Prenatal Diagnosis: Cases & Clinical Challenges

Prenatal Diagnosis: Cases & Clinical Challenges

Miriam S. DiMaio
MSW
Senior Genetic Counselor
Department of Genetics
Yale University School of Medicine
New Haven, CT
USA

Joyce E. Fox
MD
Chief, Division of Medical Genetics
Schneider Children's Hospital
Professor of Clinical Pediatrics
Albert Einstein College of Medicine
New Hyde Park, NY
USA

Maurice J. Mahoney
MD, JD
Professor of Genetics, Pediatrics, Obstetrics,
Gynecology and Reproductive Sciences
Department of Genetics
Yale University School of Medicine
New Haven, CT
USA

⊗WILEY-BLACKWELL

A John Wiley & Sons, Ltd., Publication

This edition first published 2010, © 2010 by Miriam S. DiMaio, Joyce E. Fox and Maurice J. Mahoney

Blackwell Publishing was acquired by John Wiley & Sons in February 2007. Blackwells publishing program has been merged with Wiley's global Scientific, Technical and Medical business to form Wiley-Blackwell.

Registered office: John Wiley & Sons Ltd, The Atrium, Southern Gate, Chichester, West Sussex, PO19 8SQ, UK

Editorial offices: 9600 Garsington Road, Oxford, OX4 2DQ, UK
                       The Atrium, Southern Gate, Chichester, West Sussex, PO19 8SQ, UK
                       111 River Street, Hoboken, NJ 07030-5774, USA

For details of our global editorial offices, for customer services and for information about how to apply for permission to reuse the copyright material in this book please see our website at www.wiley.com/wiley-blackwell

The right of the author to be identified as the author of this work has been asserted in accordance with the Copyright, Designs and Patents Act 1988.

ISBN: 9781405191432

A catalogue record for this book is available from the British Library and the Library of Congress.

Set in 9.25/11.5pt Minion by Thomson Digital, Noida, India

Printed and bound in Malaysia by Vivar Printing Sdn Bhd

01   2010

Contents

Preface

The advent of mid-trimester amniocentesis in the mid-1960s initiated the era of prenatal diagnosis, a new window into fetal development, health and disease. At that time, the molecular basis of almost all Mendelian disorders was unknown, and few genetic disorders could be tested for prenatally. Initially, fetal diagnosis was largely restricted to chromosomal abnormalities, the few single gene disorders for which molecular or biochemical testing could be performed on amniocytes or amniotic fluid supernatant, and fetal abnormalities that could be identified by ultrasound examination. For some rare disorders, more invasive and riskier testing by fetal blood or skin sampling or fetoscopy could provide information about the fetus.

In the ensuing decades, the explosion of knowledge about the human genome and the molecular pathogenesis of many human diseases, the availability of rapid and highly accurate molecular diagnostic techniques, and the refinement of ultrasound imaging techniques have transformed the field of prenatal diagnosis. Furthermore, maternal serum analyte testing and carrier screening for genetic disorders based on ethnic background, family history or population risk have improved our ability to identify women who are appropriate candidates for diagnostic testing. Next on the horizon will be the diagnosis of fetal disease states using fetal nucleic acids (RNA or DNA) recovered from the maternal circulation. This will markedly alter the current state of prenatal diagnosis and will probably supplant many of our current approaches.

The rapid advances in understanding the molecular basis of human disease have also revealed genetic complexities and mechanisms that were only postulated or even unimagined a generation ago. We now recognize that for some disorders, different mutations in a single gene can result in markedly disparate clinical presentations. Such disorders, once defined by narrow clinical criteria, are now known to have remarkable variation in their manifestations and age of onset depending on the nature of specific mutation(s) in a single gene. Conversely, the same or similar clinical phenotype can result from mutations in more than one gene. In addition, non-Mendelian mechanisms such as uniparental disomy, trinucleotide repeat expansions, and epigenetic phenomenona such as imprinting add another level of complexity when considering an underlying diagnosis.

A problem that often complicates counseling in prenatal diagnosis is the difficulty of making precise predictions about the severity of a disorder that has been diagnosed in utero. This is most common when chromosomal mosaicism is diagnosed in chorionic villi or amniotic fluid and where the possible outcomes range from a disabling condition to normal or near normal. Counseling is also difficult for disorders which have highly variable severity among members of the same family, are of mid-life onset, have a wide range in age of onset, or have reduced penetrance.

For some fetal abnormalities diagnosed on ultrasound examination, there is insufficient information to establish a diagnosis. Questions about the etiology of the fetal abnormalities and their recurrence in subsequent children may have to be resolved after delivery following examination of the baby or by the results of pathological examination that allow a more focused approach to molecular or other testing. Sometimes, however, an underlying diagnosis will not be established, and providing precise information about risk of recurrence is not possible. Empiric data may be available and provide some guidance. Such data, however, reflect the experience of many families and represent an average risk with some families having a much higher or lower risk.

Exposure to common and unusual clinical problems in prenatal diagnosis should be an integral component in the training of obstetricians, medical geneticists, and genetic counselors. A major shortcoming of such training is that the clinical experience is usually limited to a short period of time in which few complex cases will arise. Physicians and genetic counselors in training are therefore not exposed to the broad range of diagnostic problems and dilemmas that occur in the field of prenatal diagnosis, and they finish their training programs with only superficial clinical exposure. We hope that this book will serve as a supplement to clinical training in the field of prenatal diagnosis.

This book is a product of our own clinical experience over several decades. We have used cases from our own practice and from colleagues elsewhere, some of which have been modified, and present them as vignettes to portray diagnostic problems in prenatal diagnosis. We recognize that our case material reflects predominantly the experience of prenatal diagnosis in the United States and Canada and that medical centers in other parts of the world may have a different experience. Our presentations also reflect, to some degree, protocols that have been developed at our own medical centers.

The format of the book includes a brief synopsis of each case followed by a discussion of the problem, an explanation of the underlying biology, the available testing options, and the results that might be obtained. These cases illustrate approaches to management, including pedigree interpretation, probability, laboratory and technical analysis, and counseling. This book is not a comprehensive reference about prenatal diagnosis and is not intended to provide in-depth information about the genetic disorders that are discussed. In the interest of presenting cases in a straightforward way, our discussions may lack some of the complexities and nuances that would be found in more comprehensive sources. Some of the cases presented in the book include clinical situations or laboratory results that are rarely encountered in a general prenatal genetics practice. We have chosen to use these unusual cases because they illustrate important concepts about disease causation which have applicability to other more common problems in prenatal diagnosis. As we experience the rapid changes in laboratory methods of genetic diagnosis and in imaging technology, it is easy to predict that diagnostic approaches described herein will become outdated and replaced by newer methods.

The cases emphasize three types of clinical problems which are currently the primary focus of prenatal diagnosis: chromosomal abnormalities, Mendelian disorders, and fetal structural abnormalities that can be diagnosed by ultrasound examination. Multifactorial disorders, other than those associated with structural birth defects, are neglected because their etiology is, at present, not well understood. As our understanding of the molecular and other bases of this class of disorders increases, we anticipate that there will be interest in the prenatal diagnosis of severely disabling conditions.

We have not focused on the counseling aspects of prenatal testing and the psychological impact of abnormal test results. Whether to interrupt or continue a pregnancy is one of the most wrenching decisions that a couple can face. Recognition of the different choices that parents make when confronted with the same fetal disease state reinforces the importance of impartial and non-directive counseling after a diagnosis has been established.

There are excellent web-based resources that are available and provide comprehensive information about the field. Information about many of the genetic disorders which are discussed in this book were obtained from GeneTests, which is a web based medical genetics information resource for health care providers. GeneTests provides authoritative and comprehensive peer reviewed articles that are written by experts in the field and are updated frequently. GeneTests also contains a directory of clinical and research based genetics laboratories worldwide and the genetic disorders for which testing is available. Another indispensable web based resource is Online Mendelian Inheritance in Man (OMIM), an online catalog of Mendelian traits and disorders, now numbering over 12,000 that includes their clinical presentations and underlying molecular and biochemical bases.

1 Cytogenetic Abnormalities

Introduction

The diagnosis of a common trisomy by chorionic villus sampling or amniocentesis is the most frequent reason for referral for genetic counseling in the setting of prenatal diagnosis. There is an abundance of information available in the literature about these situations to provide accurate counseling about the spectrum of structural and functional abnormalities that could be present.

This section includes cases which illustrate the challenges in counseling about several of the less common and more vexing results that can arise from prenatal diagnostic testing. Of these, chromosomal mosaicism in chorionic villi or amniotic fluid is among the most troublesome. Prenatally diagnosed chromosomal mosaicism raises the questions of whether the abnormal cell line is also present in the fetus and, if present, whether there will be fetal damage. Although further diagnostic testing can provide more information, the interpretation of additional evaluations is complicated by phenomena such as tissue-specific mosaicism, uniparental disomy, placental mosaicism with adverse effects on the placenta, fetus or both, and the lack of long-term follow-up of surviving children. Another obstacle is that each case is unique; each case has different percentages of abnormal cells in fetal tissues that make extrapolation from the experience of case reports in the literature problematic.

Structural chromosomal rearrangements also present challenges to providing definitive prognostic information. In this situation, questions about whether the normal functioning of gene(s) has been disrupted by a translocation or inversion cannot be answered satisfactorily with current testing methods. Some rearrangements involving chromosomes which have imprinted genes raise concern about uniparental disomy which must also be addressed.

Cases involving a discrepancy between the phenotypic and chromosomal sex illustrate the possibilities of laboratory error, fetal disease states, and the limitations of ultrasonographic imaging.

Uncertainties about recurrence risks are heightened when a woman has had more than one trisomic conception, raising the possibilities of gonadal mosaicism in a parent or a predisposition to non-disjunction. Finally, when a diagnosis of a trisomic fetus is made by pathologic examination alone (i.e., without karyotypic confirmation), providing definitive information about risk of recurrence is problematic. This section presents cases of both common and rare prenatally diagnosed chromosomal abnormalities to illustrate the counseling dilemmas that can arise.

Common aneuploidy – recurrence risks and counseling pitfalls

Case 1   A 38-year-old woman is referred for chorionic villus sampling; her obstetric history is remarkable for a previous pregnancy which resulted in a stillbirth of a female infant at term. The woman relates that she was told that an evaluation of the baby after delivery revealed

Prenatal Diagnosis: Cases & Clinical Challenges, 1st edition.   By Miriam S. DiMaio, Joyce E. Fox, Maurice J. Mahoney
Published 2010 by Blackwell Publishing Ltd.

trisomy 18. The woman described her baby as having clenched hands, bilateral club feet, and an absent stomach noted on a prenatal ultrasonographic examination performed shortly before delivery. The medical records were not available for review at this time.

Once a woman has had a pregnancy with trisomy 18, the risk of recurrence is about 2.5 times the risk predicted by her age at the time of next pregnancy. The risk for other aneuploidy is about 1.8 times her age-related risk after one previous trisomy 18 conception. Hypotheses that have been offered for these increased risks include gonadal mosaicism for a trisomic cell line (when there is a recurrence of the same trisomy) and a higher risk of meiotic non-disjunction (when there is a recurrence of a different trisomy). Because trisomy 18 has a low incidence, even among older women, the risk for recurrence of fetal trisomy 18 for this woman would be about 1 in 230 taking into account her age and her obstetric history. The risk for Down syndrome would be about 1 in 65. Chorionic villus sampling or amniocentesis will provide definitive information about the fetal karyotype. Alternatively, the results of first trimester screening or integrated risk assessment can incorporate the woman's a priori trisomy 18 and trisomy 21 risks based on her history into the risk assessment. Recurrence risks for common aneuploidy are discussed by Warburton *et al.* (2004).

The woman has chorionic villus sampling at 12 weeks' gestation. The karyotype of cultured chorionic villus cells is 46,XY. Ultrasonographic examination performed at 28 weeks' gestation reveals clenched hands, club feet, micrognathia, an absent stomach, and an increased amniotic fluid volume.

The fetal karyotype is normal yet the findings on ultrasonographic examination suggest a recurrence of the abnormalities seen in the patient's stillborn baby. The phenotype of trisomy 18 can sometimes mimic the fetal akinesia deformation sequence, a condition in which multiple joint contractures (arthrogryposis multiplex congenita) are present due to decreased intrauterine fetal movement. Fetal akinesia deformation sequence is an etiologically heterogeneous condition. Causes include underlying abnormalities of the central or peripheral nervous system, of muscle, of connective tissue, intrauterine vascular compromise, maternal disease states, and space constraints within the womb. Although the majority of cases are associated with low recurrence risk, some cases of fetal akinesia deformation sequence are due to an

underlying chromosomal abnormality or mutations in a gene coding for inherited disorders with autosomal dominant, autosomal recessive, X-linked, or mitochondrial inheritance.

Review of the patient's medical records is crucial to providing her with as accurate a recurrence risk as possible. Important information which should be established includes whether a chromosomal analysis was performed or whether the diagnosis of trisomy 18 was made based on physical examination alone.

The medical records from the previous pregnancy become available. The term fetus had contractures at all major joints and a small chin. The internal organs were not examined. A skin biopsy was obtained for chromosomal analysis; cells failed to grow in the laboratory and a karyotype could not be obtained. The medical record states that the differential diagnosis included trisomy 18 and the spectrum of disorders which lead to the fetal akinesia deformation sequence.

Relying on the patient's own report is hazardous in this situation. While the patient was told that trisomy 18 was a possible explanation for her baby's abnormalities, she apparently either did not remember or did not understand that other disease states were included in the differential diagnosis. Without documentation that the previous stillbirth had trisomy 18, other diagnostic entities need to be considered.

Referral for genetics evaluation is now indicated. A large number of genetic disorders can lead to the fetal akinesia deformation sequence. An extensive genetic evaluation of the baby after delivery is indicated.

Further questioning of the mother reveals that she and her husband are first cousins.

The history of consanguinity increases the likelihood that an autosomal recessive condition is the underlying basis for the etiology of the fetal abnormalities. This information can help narrow the differential diagnosis and direct the diagnostic evaluation. Even if the mode of inheritance is thought to be secure, the underlying genetic defect present in the family may not be identifiable, due to the genetic heterogeneity of this disorder. The most common autosomal recessive disorder which can present with fetal akinesia is spinal muscular atrophy due to mutations in the *SMN1* gene. The incidence of spinal muscular atrophy varies among different ethnic groups. Homozygosity for deletions of exons 7 and 8 of the *SMN1* gene are found in 95–98% of affected individuals with the remainder being compound heterozygotes for the deletion and a point mutation in the *SMN1* gene.

> *Analysis of DNA obtained from cultured amniocytes revealed that the fetus is homozygous for deletions of exons 7 and 8 in the SMN1 gene.*

> **Case 2** *A 30-year-old woman is referred for genetic counseling because she had a sister who reportedly had Down syndrome and died in the newborn period. The karyotype of the sister is not known. No other family members reportedly have Down syndrome. The woman has a healthy brother.*

The risk for having a child with Down syndrome depends on whether the sister had Down syndrome due to trisomy 21, which is the most likely situation, or to an unbalanced inherited chromosomal translocation which may be carried by this patient in the balanced form.

About 95% of cases of Down syndrome are due to trisomy 21. Unaffected siblings of individuals with trisomy 21 Down syndrome do not have an increased risk of having a child with a chromosomal abnormality. About 4% of individuals with Down syndrome have an unbalanced Robertsonian translocation usually involving chromosome 21 and another acrocentric chromosome (13;21, 14;21, 15;21, 21;22, 21;21 translocations). Unbalanced Robertsonian translocations associated with Down syndrome arise de novo in about two-thirds of cases and the rest are inherited from a parent.

Women who carry Robertsonian translocations involving chromosome 21 have a 10–15% chance of having a fetus with Down syndrome who survives into the second trimester or beyond. The risk of a viable fetus with Down syndrome due to an unbalanced Robertsonian translocation involving chromosome 21 is less than 1% when the translocation is transmitted by a father who is a balanced carrier. Although the risk that our patient carries a Robertsonian translocation is small, definitive information is only available by establishing her peripheral blood karyotype. Array CGH (comparative genomic hybridization) would not provide useful information for this woman because this methodology identifies deletions and duplications of genetic material but does not identify balanced structural rearrangements.

There are some features in a pedigree that heighten concern about a chromosomal rearrangement segregating in a family. These include more than one affected family member with mental retardation and birth defects (or Down syndrome in the case of Robertsonian translocations involving chromosome 21), stillbirths, recurrent pregnancy loss, and subfertility or infertility. These latter problems reflect the decreased viability of chromosomally abnormal conceptuses.

> **Case 3** *The results of amniocentesis for a 39-year-old woman indicate that the fetus has trisomy 18 (47,XX,+18). Her obstetric history is remarkable for an intrauterine fetal demise at 33 weeks in a fetus who had trisomy 18 diagnosed at 28 weeks' gestation after ultrasonographic examination revealed severe intrauterine growth retardation and congenital heart disease. She was 33 years of age. She also has a healthy son. All pregnancies have been with her husband. No other relatives have had children with birth defects, recurrent miscarriages, or late fetal deaths.*

This is the second conception of a fetus with trisomy 18 in this woman. Understanding the reason for the recurrence and predicting a risk for still another occurrence are both unsatisfactory. The two occurrences could be by chance alone given that the woman is 39 years old and is at significant risk for fetal aneuploidy. A second explanation is low-grade mosaicism for trisomy 18 in one member of the couple. The mosaicism would involve an unknowable percentage of germline cells (sperm or ova) and might be demonstrable in peripheral blood lymphocytes or other cell types. There are a small number of persons with identified mosaicism reported in the literature. A third hypothesis raises the possibility of some factor (genetic or otherwise) that increases the rate of meiotic non-disjunction.

Further reading

1 Hook EB, Cross PK, Jackson L *et al.* (1988) Maternal age-specific rate of 47,+21 and other cytogenetic abnormalities diagnosed in the first trimester of pregnancy in chorionic villus biopsy specimens: comparison with rates expected from observations at amniocentesis. *American Journal of Human Genetics* **42**(6):797–807.

2 Snijders RJM, Holzgreve W, Cuckle H *et al.* (1994) Maternal age-specific risk for trisomies at 9–14 weeks gestation. *Prenatal Diagnosis* **14**:543–552.

3 Snijders RJ, Sundberg K, Holzgreve W *et al.* (1999) Maternal age- and gestation-specific risk for trisomy 21. *Ultrasound in Obstetrics and Gynecology* **13**:167–170.

4 Warburton D, Dallaire L, Thangavelu M *et al.* (2004) Trisomy recurrence: a reconsideration based on North American data. *American Journal of Human Genetics* **75** (3):376–385.

Reciprocal translocations and structural abnormalities

Case 1 *A healthy 39-year-old woman had amniocentesis at 16 weeks' gestation due to maternal age. Her husband is also 39 years old and healthy. The couple has had three early miscarriages without information about the chromosomal status of the conceptions. The amniocyte metaphase karyotype revealed an "apparently balanced" translocation between part of the short arm of chromosome 3 and part of the long arm of chromosome 7 [46,XY, t(3;7)(p13.1;q31.2)]. Ultrasonographic examination performed at the time of amniocentesis revealed normal fetal anatomy. The family histories of the patient and her husband were unremarkable for birth defects, mental retardation, classic genetic disease, stillbirths, or miscarriages.*

Balanced chromosomal rearrangements are found in a few percent of phenotypically normal individuals who have experienced recurrent spontaneous pregnancy loss. When a woman has had two or three miscarriages, chromosomal analysis of both members of the couple should be performed.

The chromosomal translocation found in the amniotic fluid cells raises concerns about associated damage to the fetus because one or both of the breakpoints could disrupt normal functioning of gene(s) at or near the sites of the breaks. In addition, there might be missing or extra genetic material at the breakpoints that cannot be detected by visual inspection of the chromosomes under the light microscope. An "apparently balanced" chromosomal rearrangement (a translocation or inversion) may therefore actually be associated with duplications or deletions of genetic material. In fact, apparently balanced chromosomal rearrangements are overrepresented in individuals with mental retardation and birth defects, confirming the limitations of routine chromosomal analysis by light microscopy.

A prenatally diagnosed apparently balanced chromosomal rearrangement may have arisen as a de novo event in the sperm or ovum, or may have been transmitted from either the mother or father who carries the same translocation in their somatic and gonadal tissues. The risk of adverse effects on fetal development will depend on whether the translocation is present constitutionally in one of the parents. Therefore, the next step is to establish the peripheral blood karyotypes of both parents.

Scenario 1 *The father's peripheral blood karyotype appears identical to that of the fetus: [46,XY,t(3p13.1;7q31.2)].*

Inherited chromosomal rearrangements involving two chromosomal breakpoints are not associated with a significantly increased risk of birth defects. In this scenario, we have also found the translocation in the 39-year-old father who is in good health. This provides reassurance that the translocation is unlikely to be disrupting crucial genes in him or to be associated with clinically important extra or missing genetic material.

While we can be reassuring that the fetus is unlikely to suffer clinical consequences as a result of the translocation, there are circumstances where two members of the same family have the same "apparently balanced" chromosomal rearrangement but have discordant phenotypes. It is important to acknowledge these unlikely possibilities and why they might occur.

There a number of different reasons which could explain how two individuals in the same family with the same apparently balanced translocation would have different phenotypes.

1 The discordant phenotypes could reflect subtle differences in the translocation (i.e., a duplication or deletion) that occurred during meiosis that could not be detected by routine cytogenetic studies.

2 The translocation might have disrupted a recessive gene in the parent which is compensated for by a normal gene on the chromosomal homolog. For example, in this case, one of the father's breakpoints is at the cystic fibrosis (*CFTR* gene) locus on chromosome 7. If this were the case, the father is unaffected by cystic fibrosis because his other *CFTR* gene (on his homologous chromosome 7) is normal. However, the fetus inherits another chromosome 7 homolog *from his mother*. If the mother's *CFTR* gene on this chromosome has a mutation, the fetus would have cystic fibrosis symptoms after birth due to the presence of two cystic fibrosis mutations.

3 The father is only 39 years old. Whether the gene(s) involved in the breakpoints of his chromosomal translocation are associated with later-onset disorders is not known.

4 Other genetic or epigenetic influences on genes affected by the translocation, e.g., imprinting, may be present.

To assess the risk of cystic fibrosis, CFTR gene mutation screening or CFTR gene sequencing of the parents and DNA obtained from cultured amniocytes are available, if desired by the couple.

Experience with array CGH in the prenatal diagnosis setting is still limited at the present time. This analysis has the potential to detect chromosomal deletions and insertions that are below the resolution of the metaphase karyotype. Interpretation of array CGH analysis can be complicated by the finding of DNA variants of uncertain clinical importance.

The finding of the translocation in the father also has implications for future pregnancies. The father produces sperm with normal, balanced, and unbalanced amounts of genetic material depending on the segregation of the chromosomes during meiosis. Thus, the couple may face an increased risk of fertility problems due to the chromosomal translocation.

The fertility problems that may occur when a parent has a balanced chromosomal rearrangement include difficulty with conception and recurrent miscarriage occurring due to chromosomally unbalanced concep-tuses arising from the rearrangement found in the father, and the increased risk of segmental uniparental disomy (for discussion of uniparental disomy see section on Robertsonian translocations).

The chance of an unbalanced viable fetus that survives into later pregnancy or after birth is also increased. Predictions about the likelihood of subfertility or chro-mosomally unbalanced viable conceptions depend on the size of the unbalanced products of the translocation and the reproductive history of the couple. Identification of the translocation in other family members and their reproductive experience may also help with predictions. In addition, there may be "interchromosomal effects" of the translocation during meiosis in which the transloca-tion interferes with normal pairing of other chromo-somes, leading to an increased risk of aneuploidy.

Prenatal diagnosis by chorionic villus sampling or amniocentesis can address the risk of a fetus with an unbalanced translocation or with aneuploidy. Preimplan-tation genetic diagnosis could also be utilized to identify embryos with unbalanced translocations and introduce only chromosomally normal or balanced embryos to the womb.

The translocation in the father may have been inherited from one of his parents or arisen de novo in the sperm or egg with which he was conceived. If one of his parents is also a translocation carrier, each of the father's siblings has a significant chance of carrying the translocation. This information would be important to share with the father's siblings so they can be counseled about possible fertility problems and an increased risk of birth defects.

Scenario 2 *The karyotypes of both parents are normal. Non-paternity is denied by the patient.*

Prospective identification and follow-up of other preg-nancies with apparently balanced de novo chromosomal rearrangements (translocations and inversions) indicates that risks of obvious birth defects are increased two- to threefold over the background risk of 3% faced by the general population. These increased risks presumably represent unbalanced genetic rearrangements that cannot be ascertained by chromosome analysis. There has been no specific pattern of birth defects in the abnormal fetuses and newborns that have been studied. Risks of learning/behavioral difficulties have not been assessed because there is very limited long-term follow-up of children with de novo apparently balanced chromosomal rearrange-ments. Because structural birth defects are increased, associated neurodevelopmental problems are also likely.

Array CGH of fetal DNA (obtained from cultured amniocytes or chorionic villi) can detect some deletions and duplications of genetic material that are below the resolution of the light microscope. Array CGH may also be necessary on the parents' DNA because interpretation of array CGH analysis can be complicated by the finding of DNA variants of uncertain clinical importance. The turnaround time for obtaining results should influence decisions about whether testing of the parents' samples should be done simultaneously with that of the fetus.

Detailed ultrasonographic examination and fetal echo-cardiography should be performed to look for anatomic abnormalities in the fetus. It is estimated that about one-third of the defects associated with de novo chro-mosomal rearrangements would be detectable by prenatal sonography.

Case 2 *A couple is referred for genetic counseling to discuss the results of amniocentesis. The amniocyte kar-yotype is 46,XY,del(13)(q12q14). This is an unbalanced chromosomal complement in which there is an interstitial deletion of a proximal segment of the long arm of chromosome 13. Array CGH shows a 13 MB deletion including deletion of the retinoblastoma gene. The pe-ripheral blood karyotypes of both members of the couple are normal.*

Small deletions of the long arm of chromosome 13 are a rare chromosomal finding and there are only a few case reports of affected individuals. The phenotype described from the case reports includes growth retardation, facial dysmorphology (frontal bossing, bulbous tip of the nose, thick lower lip, large ears and lobes), and mild to moderate mental retardation. Hydrocephalus and neurologic abnormalities may also be part of the phenotype. Absence of one copy of the retinoblastoma gene is predictive of significant increase in risk of malignancy.

Risk of recurrence of another child with a chromosome 13q deletion is small, although higher than that for other couples in the general population. The small increase in risk reflects the unlikely possibility that one of the parents carries a chromosomal rearrangement or an interstitial deletion involving chromosome 13 in their gonadal cells. The fetal karyotype could be established by chorionic villus sampling beginning at 10 weeks' gestation in a future pregnancy if the couple desired early prenatal diagnosis. Ultrasonographic examination has little, if any, utility in the diagnosis of this chromosomal abnormality.

Further reading

1 De Braekeleer M, Dao T-N (1990) Cytogenetic studies in couples experiencing repeated pregnancy losses. *Human Reproduction* **5**:519–528.

2 Gardner RJM, Sutherland GR (2004) *Chromosome Abnormalities and Genetic Counseling*, 3rd edition. Oxford University Press.

3 Warburton D (1991) De novo balanced chromosome rearrangements and extra marker chromosomes identified at prenatal diagnosis: clinical significance and distribution of breakpoints. *American Journal of Human Genetics* **49**:995–1013.

Robertsonian translocations

Case 1 *A healthy 31-year-old woman is referred for genetic counseling. After having one healthy child, she had three miscarriages in early pregnancy. All her pregnancies have been with the same partner. Her husband's peripheral blood karyotype is normal (46,XY). She has a balanced Robertsonian translocation between chromosomes 14 and 21 [45,XX,der(14q;21q)].*

Constitutional balanced chromosomal rearrangements, which are seen in about 1 in 400 phenotypically normal individuals, are associated with an increased risk of spontaneous pregnancy loss, chromosomally unbalanced liveborns, and occasionally, infertility. Empiric data suggest that after three or more miscarriages, the probability that one member of a couple has a balanced chromosomal rearrangement, either a chromosomal translocation or chromosomal inversion, is 3–5%. Identification of a balanced chromosomal rearrangement in an individual provides the couple with the likely explanation for their fertility problems, forewarns them about the possibility of a liveborn with an unbalanced chromosomal rearrangement, and affords them the opportunity for preimplantation or prenatal genetic diagnosis.

Robertsonian translocations refer to a specific class of chromosomal rearrangements in which there is fusion of the long arms of two acrocentric chromosomes (chromosomes 13, 14, 15, 21, and 22). Robertsonian translocations can be homologous in which there is fusion of the long arms of the same acrocentric chromosome, or nonhomologous, i.e., fusion of the long arms of two different acrocentric chromosomes. Balanced Robertsonian translocations are the most common human chromosomal translocation with an incidence of 1 in 900 (Table 1.1). About 4% of liveborns with Down syndrome are due to unbalanced Robertsonian translocations involving chromosome 21.

The large majority of Robertsonian translocations are between non-homologous acrocentric chromosomes, and the 13;14 Robertsonian translocation is the most common.

The short arm of an acrocentric chromosome is comprised of the satellite, the satellite stalk, and the proximal short arm. The satellite stalk, also known as the nucleolar organizing region, contains multiple copies of genes coding for ribosomal RNA. An individual with one Robertsonian translocation has only eight satellite stalks instead of the usual ten. However, this reduction is not detrimental although, presumably, a minimum number of stalks with active genes is necessary for normal cellular function.

Table 1.1 Robertsonian translocations

Non-homologous Robertsonian translocations			
t(13;14)*	t(14;15)	t(15;21)**	t(21;22)**
t(13;15)	t(14;21)**	t(15;22)	
t(13;21)**	t(14;22)		
t(13;22)			
Homologous Robertsonian translocations			
t(13;13)			
t(14;14)			
t(15;15)			
t(21;21)**			
t(22;22)			

*Most common, **less common, remainder very rare.

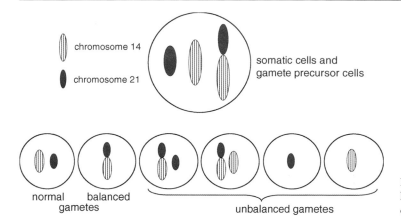

Figure 1.1 Meiotic segregation in the non-homologous Robertsonian translocation carrier.

With rare exceptions, balanced Robertsonian translocations are not associated with adverse effects on health or development. Individuals with balanced Robertsonian translocations do have an increased risk of infertility, recurrent spontaneous abortions, and, depending on the chromosomes involved in the translocation, an increased risk of chromosomally unbalanced viable fetuses and children. These problems occur because the Robertsonian translocation causes abnormal segregation of the chromosomes during meiosis, resulting in gametes with six different possible chromosomal configurations, only two of which are balanced, as shown in Figure 1.1. Thus, at fertilization, the zygote could have an entirely normal chromosomal complement, the balanced translocation, or various combinations of unbalanced products as illustrated in Figure 1.2.

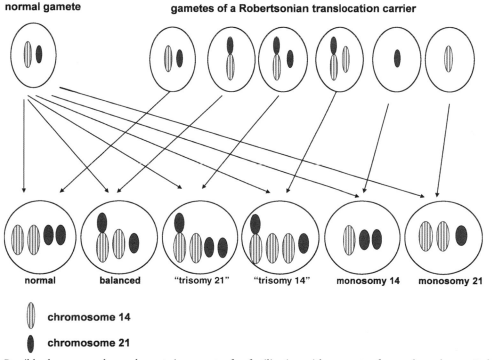

Figure 1.2 Possible chromosomal complements in a zygote after fertilization with a gamete of a non-homologous Robertsonian translocation carrier.

The risk that a balanced Robertsonian translocation carrier will have a viable chromosomally unbalanced fetus at the time of amniocentesis or later in pregnancy is shown in Table 1.2. Although two-thirds of zygotes shown in Figure 1.2 are chromosomally unbalanced, most fetuses of Robertsonian translocation carriers – i.e., all the monosomic fetuses, most fetuses who have three copies of chromosomes 13, and virtually all fetuses with three copies of chromosomes 14, 15, or 22 – will not survive for more than a few days or weeks following fertilization. This accounts for the overall low risk of viable unbalanced fetuses among parents who carry a non-homologous Robertsonian translocation.

The risk of unbalanced embryos surviving into the second trimester or after birth depends on the chromosomes involved in the translocation and which parent carries the Robertsonian translocation. As shown in Table 1.2, the risk is highest for women who carry a

Table 1.2 Frequency of unbalanced translocations at the time of amniocentesis* in non-homologous Robertsonian translocation carriers

Robertsonian translocation	Balanced carrier mother: % unbalanced at amniocentesis	Balanced carrier father: % unbalanced at amniocentesis
13q14q	1	<1
13q15q	1	<1
13q21q	10–15	<1
13q22q	1	<1
14q15q	0	0
14q21q	10–15	<1
14q22q	0	0
15q21q	10–15	<1
15q22q	<1	<1

*Frequency at livebirth is less than in the second trimester.
Estimates for rare Robertsonian translocations are extrapolated from data for the common Robertsonian translocations.
Risk of uniparental disomy 14 or 15 is about 0.65% (CI 0.2–2.3%) for Robertsonian translocations involving chromosomes 14 and 15. Carriers of homologous Robertsonian translocations (13q13q, 14q14q, 15q15q, 21q21q, 22q;22q) have a remote chance of having a chromosomally normal conceptus because their gametes will either be nullisomic or disomic for the translocation chromosome. Monosomy for other than the X chromosome results in embryonic death. Trisomy for chromosomes 14 and 15 results in early embryonic death. Fetuses with trisomy for chromosomes 13 or 22 rarely survive into the early second trimester or beyond. 21q21q homologous translocation carriers have a significant risk of a viable fetus with trisomy 21.
Data adapted from Gardner and Sutherland (2004) and Silverstein *et al.* (2002).

non-homologous Robertsonian translocation involving chromosome 21. For 14;21 and 21;22 translocation carriers, the risk at the time of amniocentesis of a viable fetus with Down syndrome is about 15% for a female Robertsonian translocation carrier. In contrast, this risk is only about 1% for a male Robertsonian translocation carrier. The significantly lower risk of viable chromosomally unbalanced fetuses in pregnancies where the father transmits a Robertsonian translocation involving chromosome 21 might reflect selection against chromosomally unbalanced sperm during gametogenesis or fertilization. In contrast to the high risk of Down syndrome in fetuses of women with Robertsonian translocations involving chromosome 21, individuals with non-homologous Robertsonian translocations involving chromosome 13, regardless of their sex, have only a small chance of having a fetus with three copies of chromosome 13 who survives into the second trimester of pregnancy. Individuals with non-homologous Robertsonian translocations involving chromosomes other than 13 and 21 have a very small risk of having a viable fetus with a non-mosaic trisomy even late in the first trimester.

Some individuals with balanced non-homologous Robertsonian translocations experience recurrent early pregnancy loss while others do not. These variations may exist even between members of the same family and do not have a satisfactory explanation. Preimplantation genetic diagnosis might be considered for a couple who have had recurrent miscarriages with unbalanced fetuses.

Due to their rarity, no empiric data are available about the risks of viable unbalanced fetuses for individuals who carry 13;21 and 15;21 Robertsonian translocations. However, we believe the reproductive experience probably would parallel that of the carriers of 14;21 and 21;22 Robertsonian translocations as shown in Table 1.2.

The risk of birth defects in the balanced offspring of a parent who has a balanced Robertsonian translocation involving chromosome 14 (i.e., 13;14; 14;15; 14;21; 14;22), chromosome 15 (i.e., 13;15; 14;15; 15;21; 15;22), and 21;22 is slightly increased over the 3% background risk of birth defects. The slight increase in risk reflects phenomena such as uniparental disomy with imprinting, expression of a recessive gene, or underlying mosaicism in the fetus for a cell line which is trisomic due to an unbalanced Robertsonian translocation.

Uniparental disomy refers to the possibility that the diploid cell line, the "normal" cells, has both of its number 14 or number 15 chromosomes coming from one parent. This arises when early in embryogenesis a trisomic conceptus (trisomy 14 or 15) is "rescued" from embryonic death by a non-disjunction event resulting in loss of one of the number 14 or 15 chromosomes. Both maternal and paternal uniparental disomy 14 and 15 are associated with deleterious effects on normal development. Maternal disomy for chromosome 14 has effects on development of variable severity including prenatal and postnatal growth restriction and facial dysmorphology. Cognitive functioning ranges from normal to severe retardation. Paternal disomy 14 is associated with polyhydramnios, prenatal and postnatal growth restriction, a small thorax, and kyphosis. Maternal disomy 15 is one mechanism that leads to Prader–Willi syndrome and paternal disomy 15 to Angelman syndrome. There is no evidence for deleterious effects of maternal or paternal imprinting of genes on chromosomes 13, 21, and 22 as neither maternal nor paternal uniparental disomy for these chromosomes has been associated with an abnormal phenotype.

In addition to trisomy rescue two other recognized mechanisms, gamete complementation and gamete compensation, can lead to uniparental disomy. Gamete complementation occurs when an ovum missing a specific chromosome is fertilized by a sperm which by chance has two copies of that same chromosome. Gamete compensation refers to the situation where a zygote which is monosomic for a certain chromosome is rescued from embryonic death by a mitotic nondisjunction event leading to duplication of that chromosome.

When a parent carries a Robertsonian translocation involving chromosomes 14 or 15, the risk of uniparental disomy is about 0.65% (95% CI 0.2–2.3%).

Uniparental disomy may cause problems in the fetus due to the presence of recessive alleles or deletions at a gene locus or due to the effects of genetic imprinting. Imprinting refers to the situation in which genes behave differently depending on whether they are inherited from the mother or the father. For example, some genes will only be expressed on a maternally inherited chromosome and others only on a paternally inherited chromosome. For some, but not all genes, absence of a maternal or paternal contribution will result in adverse effects on development or function. Chromosomes containing genes which are imprinted and the clinical consequences of imprinting are listed in Table 1.3.

Trisomy rescue during embryogenesis can also lead to the situation in which a fetus is mosaic for a disomic and a chromosomally unbalanced cell line. Phenotypic effects are highly variable and depend on the percentage and distribution of the chromosomally abnormal cells. Chorionic villus sampling or amniocentesis should identify most situations in which the fetus has a large percentage of chromosomally unbalanced cells. Low-level mosaicism, however, may go undetected. The experience with prenatal diagnosis with Robertsonian translocation carriers indicates that if the chorionic villus or amniocyte karyotype is normal, the probability of deleterious underlying mosaicism for a chromosomally unbalanced cell line is very small.

Testing for whole chromosome uniparental disomy 14 or 15 can be accomplished by analysis of DNA obtained from chorionic villi or amniocytes and the peripheral blood cells of the parents. DNA polymorphisms associated with the specific chromosome are analyzed to determine whether there is chromosomal material from both parents. Detection of some cases of uniparental disomy is also becoming available by analysis of the fetal DNA alone.

Case 2 Chromosomal analysis is performed on a newborn after a pediatrician suspects that he has Down syndrome. The karyotype of the baby is 46,XY,-21,+t(21q;21q). The baby has Down syndrome because he has a homologous Robertsonian translocation involving chromosome 21 with two copies of chromosome 21 genes, in addition to a free-standing chromosome 21. Analysis of the parents' peripheral blood karyotypes is indicated.

Available data show that 90% of unbalanced homologous Robertsonian translocations causing Down syndrome arise as de novo events. In 10% of cases, one of the parents is found to carry the homologous Robertsonian translocation. Homologous translocations for the other acrocentric chromosomes in fetuses are very rare and the percentage of those arising de novo is not known.

If the translocation has arisen de novo in the baby, the risk of recurrence is very small, only slightly increased over the background risk faced by all couples. This slightly increased risk reflects the unlikely possibility that one of the parents has mosaicism for the homologous Robertsonian translocation in his or her germ cells.

If a parent carries the translocation, the chance of having a chromosomally normal child is remote. The gametes of the parent with the homologous Robertsonian translocation contain either two copies of chromosome 21 or no copy. The former situation results in conceptuses with three copies of chromosome 21 and the latter results in conceptuses with monosomy 21 which is lethal during early embryogenesis.

Table 1.3 Abnormal phenotypes associated with whole chromosome uniparental disomy (UPD)

Maternal UPD	Chromosome	Paternal UPD
	1	
	2	
	3	
	4	
	5	
	6	Transient neonatal diabetes, IUGR, macroglossia
Pre- and postnatal growth retardation; relative macrocephaly; facial dysmorphism resembling Russell–Silver syndrome; developmental delay in some cases, retarded bone age	7	
	8	
	9	
	10	
	11	Beckwith–Wiedemann syndrome
	12	
	13	
Pre- and postnatal growth retardation; facial dysmorphism (large and broad forehead, high palate, fleshy nasal tip, slight blepharophimosis), muscular hypotonia; precocious puberty; obesity, wide range of intellectual deficits	14	Polyhydramnios and premature labor; pre- and postnatal growth retardation; small bell-shaped thorax with short, curved ribs, kyphosis, all of variable severity
Prader–Willi syndrome	15	Angelman syndrome
	16	
	17	
	18	
	19	
	20	
	21	
	X	
	patXY	

Adapted from Kotzot D, Utermann G (2005) *American Journal of Medical Genetics* **136A**:287–305. The chromosomes with no clinical descriptions have not been associated with a clinical phenotype at this time.

There have been rare reports of chromosomally normal or chromosomally balanced children born to individuals who carry homologous Robertsonian translocations. This can be due to underlying gonadal mosaicism for a normal cell line in the carrier parent, or, by trisomy rescue, gamete compensation or gamete complementation.

Couples in which one member of the couple carries a homologous Robertsonian translocation should be counseled that the chance of a chromosomally balanced fetus is remote. Infertility, recurrent miscarriage, or in the case of individuals with 21;21 and 13;13 Robertsonian translocations, viable fetuses with Down syndrome or trisomy 13 would be expected. Pregnancy could be achieved by either egg or sperm donation.

Further reading

1 Boue A, Gallano P (1984) Collaborative study of the segregation of inherited chromosome structural rearrangements in 1356 prenatal diagnoses. *Prenatal Diagnosis* **4**:45–67.
2 Cox H, Bullman H, Temple IK (2004) Maternal UPD (14) in the patient with a normal karyotype: clinical report and systematic search for case in samples sent for testing for Prader–Willi syndrome. *American Journal of Medical Genetics* **127A**:21–25.
3 Daniel A, Hook EB, Wulf G (1989) Risks of unbalanced progeny at amniocentesis to carriers of chromosome rearrangements: data from United States and Canadian laboratories. *American Journal of Human Genetics* **33** (1):14–53.

4 Gardner RJ, Sutherland GR (2004) *Chromosome Abnormalities and Genetic Counseling*, 3rd edition. Oxford University Press.

5 Kotzot D, Utermann G (2005) Uniparental disomy (UPD) other than 15: phenotypes and bibliography updated. *American Journal of Medical Genetics* **136** (3):287–305.

6 Silverstein S, Lerer I, Sagi M *et al.* (2002) Uniparental disomy in fetuses diagnosed with balanced Robertsonian translocations: risk estimate. *Prenatal Diagnosis* **22** (8):649–651.

Chromosomal mosaicism – prenatal diagnosis

Chromosomal mosaicism refers to the situation in which there are cells with different chromosomal complements. It may occur in an individual or in the in vitro culture of cells in a laboratory sample. In liveborns, there is a phenotypic continuum associated with chromosomal mosaicism which ranges from normal or near normal to the classic manifestations of the chromosomal abnormality. Chromosomal mosaicism is often found in amniotic fluid and chorionic villus cell culture. How we determine whether chromosomally abnormal cells found in chorionic villi or amniotic fluid pose a significant risk of underlying mosaicism in fetal tissues will be illustrated by the following cases.

The clinical importance of prenatally diagnosed chromosomal mosaicism depends on a number of factors including the level of mosaicism and the chromosomal abnormality involved.

Three levels of prenatally diagnosed chromosomal mosaicism are defined as follows.

• *Level I mosaicism* (single cell pseudomosaicism): a single abnormal cell in an otherwise normal study.

• *Level II mosaicism* (multiple cell pseudomosaicism): the presence of two or more abnormal cells with the same abnormality, which are restricted to a single culture vessel.

• *Level III mosaicism* (true mosaicism): the presence of abnormal cells with the same abnormality which are found in different culture vessels. True mosaicism means that the abnormal cell line is very unlikely to have arisen in cell culture after chorionic villus sampling or amniocentesis was performed. This conclusion is warranted because the same chromosomal abnormality is present in cells recovered from different culture vessels into which the original, uncultured sample had been placed.

Table 1.4 summarizes relevant information when considering the diagnostic problem of prenatally diagnosed chromosomal mosaicism.

Mosaicism in amniotic fluid for a common chromosomal abnormality (trisomy 21)

A woman elected amniocentesis based on her age of 35 years. The amniocyte karyotype is 47,XX,+21/46,XX. Cells with trisomy 21 are recovered from three different cover slips. About 20% of the cells have trisomy 21.

Because cells with a trisomy 21 karyotype were recovered from more than one culture vessel, level III mosaicism (true mosaicism) is present in this study.

Follow-up of pregnancies in which chromosomal mosaicism has been observed in cultured amniocytes suggests that the chromosomal mosaicism may be confined to cells shed from the placenta without phenotypic effects in the fetus. Amniotic fluid cells originate from both the fetus and the placenta although placentally derived cells are a small minority. Nonetheless, abnormal cells recovered in an amniotic fluid sample could be restricted to those originating in the placenta or membranes. Follow-up of pregnancies in which level III (true) mosaicism has been observed in amniotic fluid cells indicate a 70% or higher chance of mosaicism subsequently being confirmed in the fetus, or in the baby after birth. Predictions about the likelihood of demonstrable abnormalities that are associated with the abnormal cells are more difficult to make.

Caution must be exercised when counseling about the overall published concordance rate between amniotic fluid cell mosaicism and the underlying fetal karyotype because the above concordance rate of 70% underestimates the likelihood of a population of abnormal cells in the fetus. Follow-up studies of prenatally diagnosed cases of chromosomal mosaicism have relied mostly on an analysis of peripheral blood cells (and occasionally skin cells) of a liveborn baby or of skin cells from an aborted fetus. This is a major limitation of these studies because mosaicism for rare trisomies (e.g., trisomy 15 – see case below) is often restricted to certain somatic tissues and may be selected against in tissues that are usually submitted for cytogenetic analysis. In addition, the follow-up reports of the liveborns usually discuss the phenotypes present in the newborn period or early infancy. Later-onset developmental problems would not be recognized or reported in the literature. Thus, in the setting of an amniotic fluid study with level III mosaicism for trisomy 21, the likelihood of underlying mosaicism in the fetus is *at least* 70% and probably higher.

Further testing of the pregnancy to provide more information about the fetal karyotype could be obtained by fetal blood sampling and fetal skin biopsy. In contrast to

Table 1.4 Prenatally diagnosed chromosomal mosaicism

I Definitions
Level I mosaicism (single cell pseudomosaicism): a single abnormal cell in an otherwise normal study
Level II mosaicism (multiple cell pseudomosaicism): two or more cells with the same chromosomal abnormality in a single culture vessel or colony, or one entire colony; the abnormality is not found in cells from other culture vessels
Level III mosaicism (true mosaicism): two or more cells with the same chromosomal abnormality distributed in two or more culture vessels

	Amniocentesis	Chorionic villus sampling
II Incidence of mosaicism		
All levels	5%	>5%
Level III mosaicism	0.25%	1%
III Confirmation of mosaicism in fetus or baby		
Levels I and II	Unknown, but infrequent[#]	Unknown, but infrequent
Level III mosaicism	70%[*]	40%[*]

IV Factors influencing assessment of risk to fetus/pregnancy and recommendations, if any, for further testing
   1 Level of mosaicism and adequacy of the study
   2 Chromosomal abnormality involved
   3 Potential for phenotypic expression of uniparental disomy
   4 Phenomenon of tissue-limited mosaicism
   5 Association of confined placental mosaicism with increased risk of poor pregnancy outcome

V Options for further testing
   1 Amniocentesis after mosaicism found at CVS or repeat amniocentesis
   2 Fetal blood sampling
   3 Fetal skin biopsy
   4 Uniparental disomy studies if amniocytes are diploid
   5 Interphase cell analysis by FISH
   6 Targeted ultrasonographic examination including fetal echocardiography
   7 Chromosome studies in the newborn or infant periods

[#]Very few attempts have been made to perform postnatal cytogenetic studies in level I and level II cases to look for evidence of mosaicism; no excess risk of pregnancy loss or birth defects has been reported in this group; no long-term follow-up is available; anecdotal reports exist of level I and II prenatal mosaic findings subsequently being associated with recovery of the abnormal cell line from liveborns.
[*]Represents overall risk of all aneuploidies; actual risk in a given pregnancy must take into the account specific aneuploidy which is present.

amniocytes, which may contain a mixture of fetal and placental cells, there is no ambiguity about the origin of cells obtained from fetal blood or skin. If the fetal lymphocyte karyotype is normal, the risk of clinically important mosaicism will be significantly reduced, to a few percent or less. However, normal results of invasive testing cannot completely exclude the possibility of underlying mosaicism in the fetus as the abnormal cell line has a chance of being present in fetal tissues, such as the brain or heart, which are not sampled either before or after birth.

Although some association may exist, correlations between the percentage of abnormal cells recovered in amniocytes or a fetal tissue and the severity of effects on normal development must be made cautiously. It is impossible to know the percentage of abnormal cells in critical body organs.

Detailed ultrasonographic imaging including fetal echocardiography is recommended. The identification of anatomic or growth problems in the fetus, regardless of the results of further invasive testing of the pregnancy, will further raise concerns that the fetus has a significant fraction of abnormal cells. However, normal fetal imaging cannot significantly diminish the risk of clinically underlying mosaicism in the fetus. Even in the non-mosaic form, only about half of fetuses with Down syndrome have detectable signs on ultrasonographic examination. In the setting of mosaicism, in which a normal cell line will moderate or minimize the Down syndrome phenotype, the likelihood of visible anatomic variants or defects is even smaller. It is also important to recognize that a sonographic abnormality might have a totally independent cause unassociated with the mosaicism.

Maternal cell contamination of amniotic fluid is extremely unlikely in the cytogenetics laboratory when the amniocentesis has been uncomplicated and the first few milliliters of fluid are not used for the cytogenetic studies.

When there is no sonographic evidence at the time of amniocentesis of a co-twin, now deceased, who was noted on a first-trimester ultrasonographic examination, cells from the vanishing twin have a very low chance of being present in the amniotic fluid sample.

If the pregnancy continues to term, a karyotype could be obtained from cord blood or from peripheral blood, or from a skin biopsy in the newborn period, or no further testing be performed at all. FISH (fluorescence in situ hybridization) studies of interphase cells such as buccal mucosal cells could also be done. Normal results from testing during the pregnancy and, if desired, of the newborn would provide reasonable inference that the abnormal cell line was unassociated with adverse phenotypic effects in the fetus, but would not completely exclude them.

Mosaicism in chorionic villus cells for a rare chromosomal abnormality (trisomy 15)

A woman elected chorionic villus sampling based on her age of 40 years. The chorionic villus cell karyotype is 47, XX,+15/46,XX. Cells with trisomy 15 are found on different cover slips.

Cells with a trisomy 15 karyotype were recovered from two different initial cultures. Level III mosaicism (true mosaicism) is present in this study.

Follow-up of pregnancies in which chromosomal mosaicism has been observed in chorionic villi indicate that the chromosomal mosaicism may be confined to the placenta without phenotypic effects in the fetus. A rough estimate of its presence in the fetus is 40%.

Liveborns with birth defects have been reported who have trisomy 15 mosaicism. Recognition of the entity has been very infrequent, however. The probability of adverse phenotypic effects in the setting of chromosomal mosaicism is related to the percentage and distribution of the cells with abnormal chromosomes. Depending on the percentage and distribution of the abnormal cell line, effects could range from none or mild, to significant abnormalities including mental retardation and structural birth defects. The presence of the abnormal cell line could easily lead to early fetal death.

As with amniotic fluid cell studies, caution must be exercised when counseling about the published overall concordance rate between chorionic villus cell mosaicism and the fetal karyotype. Most studies which attempt to confirm the results of chorionic villi in a liveborn rely only on an analysis of peripheral blood cells and occasionally skin cells. In the past, most studies examined metaphase cells and did not examine interphase cells. More recent studies are including interphase cells. Especially for rare trisomies, e.g., trisomy 15, it is possible that mosaicism for the abnormal cell line is restricted to only certain fetal tissues and may be selected against in tissues that are usually submitted for cytogenetic analysis. The published studies reporting on concordance rates between mosaicism found at the time of chorionic villus sampling and subsequent recovery of abnormal cells in fetal tissue or liveborns are also limited by the fact that relatively little data are available about any specific trisomy.

Further testing of the pregnancy to provide more information about the fetal karyotype could be obtained by amniocentesis, fetal blood sampling, and fetal skin sampling. In addition to standard metaphase analysis of amniocytes, it would be useful to study the amniotic fluid cell population by FISH using a chromosome 15 probe to look for trisomy 15 cells that would not be found by metaphase analysis.

A low risk of adverse phenotypic effects will be predicted if results of amniocentesis are normal, and if detailed ultrasonographic examination documents normal fetal growth and development. However, once mosaicism has been documented in chorionic villi or amniotic fluid, normal results of further imaging or invasive testing cannot completely exclude the possibility of underlying mosaicism in the fetus as the abnormal cell line may be present in fetal tissues that cannot be sampled, and the abnormal cells may not cause an abnormal sonographic phenotype. Trisomy 15 has rarely been recovered from metaphase analysis of peripheral blood lymphocytes, suggesting that these cells may not mature in the marrow or survive in the peripheral circulation very well. In the setting of trisomy 15 mosaicism, normal results of fetal blood sampling would provide limited useful information.

If trisomy 15 cells are found in cultured amniocytes, this substantially increases the likelihood that they are populating fetal tissues. However, amniocytes are derived from both the placenta and the fetus. Recovery of trisomy 15 cells in amniotic fluid does not prove that the fetus has underlying mosaicism as the abnormal cells could still be restricted to the placenta although this subsequent finding would substantially increase the risk of true fetal mosaicism. The overall concordance rate between amniocyte mosaicism and subsequent recovery of the abnormal cells in fetal tissue or a liveborn is suggested to be about 70%. As stated earlier, this is probably an underestimate. It is likely that if trisomy 15 cells are recovered in amniotic fluid, even if ultrasonographic examination reveals normal fetal anatomy, there would be a high probability (>80%) of underlying trisomy 15 mosaicism in the fetus with a wide spectrum of possible effects.

Recovery of trisomy 15 cells from a fetal tissue, e.g., skin or blood, will further raise concerns that the fetus has a significant fraction of abnormal cells. Correlations between the percentage of abnormal cells recovered in amniocytes or a fetal tissue and the severity of effects on normal development must be made cautiously. Particularly for rare trisomies, it may not be appropriate to generalize from the karyotype of fetal lymphocytes or skin fibroblasts to other tissues such as the brain. Also, normal fetal imaging should not be used to conclude that the risk of clinically underlying mosaicism in the fetus is negligible. Karyotypically abnormal cells can have major deleterious effects on organ functioning without gross anatomic defects.

Detailed ultrasonographic imaging including fetal echocardiography is recommended. The identification of anatomic or growth problems in the fetus, regardless of the results of further invasive testing of the pregnancy, will raise concerns considerably that the fetus has suffered phenotypic effects from trisomy 15 mosaicism.

The cells with trisomy 15 could have arisen due to a chromosomal non-disjunction event which occurred in the egg or sperm with which the fetus was conceived. Alternatively, the cells with trisomy 15 could have arisen after conception by a mitotic non-disjunction event. The former explanation for the presence of the trisomy 15 cell line in chorionic villi poses some additional risk of abnormality in the fetus or placenta due to the possibility that the diploid cell line, the "normal" cells, has both of its number 15 chromosomes coming from one parent, a situation known as uniparental disomy. Uniparental disomy arises when a trisomic conceptus, trisomy 15 in this situation, is "rescued" from embryonic death by loss of one of the number 15 chromosomes to generate the mosaic condition with the diploid cell line in addition to the trisomic cell line. If there is uniparental disomy, both members of the homologous chromosome pair in the diploid cell line will have come from the same parent.

Uniparental disomy causes an abnormal phenotype due to imprinting effects or homozygosity at recessive disease loci. Recognizable genetic syndromes have been reported in association with uniparental disomy for chromosome 15 and for uniparental disomy for other chromosomes (see section on Robertsonian translocations). Prader–Willi syndrome occurs when an individual has two chromosome 15s which are maternally inherited. When both chromosome 15s are inherited from a father, this results in Angelman syndrome. Both disorders are associated with significant mental retardation, characteristic physical findings and aberrant behavior. Mosaicism due to trisomy rescue situations arise more frequently, but not exclusively, in the setting of advanced maternal age where there is an increased risk of trisomic conceptuses. The presence or absence of uniparental disomy can be established by analysis of DNA extracted from amniocytes unless there is a major fraction of trisomic cells present. Current uniparental disomy studies often require fetal DNA and DNA from both parents. New methods may make it possible to use fetal DNA only.

Unrecognized maternal cell contamination of cultured chorionic villi is a negligible problem for cytogenetic analysis when chorionic villi are expertly dissected from maternal decidua in an experienced laboratory and the cells are harvested after only a few days in culture.

For twin gestations, it is unlikely that a chorionic villus sample will be contaminated with cells from a living or deceased twin but this possibility cannot be ruled out. The obstetrician's documentation of the positional relationship of the placentas and the approach of the sampling instrument during the chorionic villus sampling procedure will be helpful in considering the likelihood of contamination.

The trisomy 15 cell line could be confined to the placenta and membranes and still pose problems for the fetus. Placental chromosomal mosaicism may lead to placental dysfunction and poor pregnancy outcome, including intrauterine growth restriction, preterm delivery and intrauterine fetal death. Even if there are no abnormal cells in the fetus, harmful effects could occur because of mosaicism in the placenta.

If the pregnancy continues to term, postnatal chromosome studies could be obtained. If they are normal, and earlier studies of the fetus had been normal, there is a reasonable inference that the abnormal cell line would be unassociated with adverse phenotypic effects in the child, although the evidence would not be conclusive.

Mosaicism in chorionic villus cells for a different rare chromosomal abnormality (trisomy 16)

The karyotype of cultured chorionic villi for a 38-year-old woman is 47,XX,+16. No cell with a normal karyotype was identified. The fetus appeared to have normal growth and development at the time of chorionic villus sampling at 12 weeks' gestation.

Trisomy 16 is one of the most common chromosomal abnormalities identified in first-trimester spontaneous miscarriages. Identification of a placenta with full or mosaic trisomy 16 is an uncommon finding. Although mosaicism with a normal cell line is not present in this case, only a small fraction of the placenta was sampled.

Liveborns with birth defects due to trisomy 16 mosaicism have been reported. This condition is very rare. Given trisomy 16 cells in the placenta, a rough estimate of its presence in the fetus is 40%. Fetal mosaicism could be associated with a wide range of anatomic and/or functional problems depending on the distribution and number of the trisomy 16 cells. From the limited literature about fetal and placental trisomy 16, up to half of fetuses would either not survive in utero or be abnormal when there is a trisomy 16 placenta. This may be due to placental insufficiency or abnormalities intrinsic to the fetus or both.

Most cases of trisomy 16 mosaicism arise following a trisomy rescue event, increasing the chance of uniparental disomy for trisomy 16. There have been a few reports of chromosomally normal infants with maternal disomy for chromosome 16. Intrauterine growth restriction has been documented in some of these cases. Rarely, birth defects or mental retardation have been present. The scarcity of cases does not allow conclusions as to whether there is a consistent pattern. It is not possible in these cases to determine whether the adverse effects on growth were attributable to imprinting problems associated with uniparental disomy, to dysfunction of a mosaic placenta, or to underlying trisomy 16 mosaicism in tissues which were not analyzed.

Further invasive testing of the pregnancy to provide more information about the fetal karyotype could be obtained by amniocentesis and fetal skin biopsy. Noninvasive testing would include detailed ultrasonographic examination including fetal echocardiography. Low risks of phenotypic effects would be predicted if results of further testing are normal and the fetus appears to have normal anatomy and growth. However, normal results of further testing cannot completely exclude the possibility of underlying mosaicism in the fetus. Trisomy 16 is rarely recovered from metaphase analysis of peripheral blood lymphocytes, suggesting that fetal blood sampling would be unlikely to provide useful information. Future studies of interphase cells in fetal blood using chromosome 16 probes may alter that conclusion, however.

Recovery of trisomy 16 cells from additional invasive testing and/or the identification of anatomic or growth problems in the fetus will considerably raise concerns that the fetus has suffered damaging effects. If growth restriction is the only finding, this might reflect an abnormal placenta with a chromosomally normal fetus. For the latter situation, there would still be uncertainty about long-term deficits for a child. Trisomy 16 cells confined to the placenta are associated with a significant risk of intrauterine growth restriction and perinatal loss.

Mosaicism in amniotic fluid for a rare chromosomal abnormality (trisomy 8)

A 37-year-old woman elects amniocentesis. The karyotype of cultured amniotic fluid cells is 46,XX. One colony contained two cells with a 47,XX,+8 karyotype. Only cells with normal karyotypes were recovered from a large number of other colonies which were examined.

Two cells with trisomy 8 from a single colony were recovered in an otherwise normal study. This is level II mosaicism (multiple cell pseudomosaicism).

Follow-up of pregnancies in which abnormal amniotic fluid cells are restricted to a single colony or culture vessel do not demonstrate an increased risk of birth defects above the background risk. These studies have significant limitations because they report the experience of level I and level II mosaicism for all chromosomal abnormalities. There is a paucity of follow-up data about mosaicism for specific chromosomes. Thus, the published studies, while reassuring, do not exclude the possibility of a small increased risk of abnormalities associated with underlying mosaicism in the fetus. Furthermore, if detrimental effects on fetal development are present, they may not be recognized at birth. There are numerous anecdotal reports of level I and level II mosaicism being associated with underlying mosaicism in the fetus or liveborn, and, at times, with adverse effects on development.

Especially for rare trisomies, e.g., trisomy 8, it is possible that mosaicism for the abnormal cell line is restricted to only certain fetal tissues and is not present in tissues that are usually submitted for cytogenetic analysis such as blood or skin.

In the setting of only two cells with trisomy 8 in an otherwise normal amniotic fluid cell study, the magnitude of risk is unknown but may be higher than for other trisomies. There are a few case reports of babies diagnosed with trisomy 8 mosaicism syndrome for whom there was only a single cell or even no abnormal cell in amniocyte culture. These reports indicate that trisomy 8 cells may not enter or survive in amniotic fluid as readily as other types of cells. The abnormalities identified in the children with trisomy 8 mosaicism but normal amniocyte karyotypes include mental retardation, cleft palate, and ophthalmologic, cardiac and renal abnormalities. Trisomy 8 mosaicism is also associated with an increased risk of hematopoietic cell malignancies.

Further testing of the pregnancy to determine whether the fetus has trisomy 8 mosaicism is complicated by the knowledge that in affected liveborns the abnormal cell line is often not present in lymphocytes. Therefore, normal results of fetal blood sampling may not be informative with respect to the possibility of underlying trisomy 8 mosaicism although studies of interphase analysis of blood cells by FISH have not been reported. Fetal skin biopsy may have the best chance of detecting trisomy 8 mosaicism if the fetus is truly mosaic. Any further cytogenetic studies should use FISH on interphase cells as well as standard metaphase analysis. If further extensive cytogenetic studies are performed and normal, there may still be a small chance of underlying trisomy 8 mosaicism in the fetus that is higher than for other chromosomes. Abnormal phenotypes have not been identified with uniparental disomy for chromosome 8.

Detailed ultrasonographic imaging including fetal echocardiography is also recommended. However, normal fetal imaging should not be used to conclude that the risk of clinically underlying mosaicism in the fetus is negligible. Karyotypically abnormal cells can have major deleterious effects on organ functioning without gross anatomic defects being present, with the brain being the most vulnerable organ. After birth, chromosome studies can be pursued from both blood and solid tissues.

General discussion on prenatally diagnosed chromosomal mosaicism

Further invasive testing of the pregnancy to provide more information about the fetal karyotype exposes the pregnancy to the risks of those procedures. Thus, whether to proceed with further invasive testing must be balanced against the likelihood of finding clinically important results that are related to underlying mosaicism in the fetus. While level III mosaicism for a numerical chromosomal abnormality raises significant concerns about underlying fetal pathology, assessing the risk of abnormalities in a fetus in the setting of level I and level II mosaicism is usually much more problematic. In experienced hands, the risk of pregnancy loss associated with fetal blood sampling and fetal skin sampling is about 1% and 3%, respectively. How to balance these procedure-related risks and the limited information they provide with the uncertain risk of fetal disease is one of the challenges faced by clinicians counseling about prenatally diagnosed mosaicism.

The decision to proceed with further invasive testing of the pregnancy should also be influenced by whether the results, normal or abnormal, will allow revision of prognosis for the fetus. For example, in the setting of level III mosaicism in amniotic fluid for the sex chromosome abnormalities, 47,XXX, 47,XXY, and 47,XYY, recovery of the abnormal cell line in fetal blood would not usually change the uncertainties of prognosis. In the setting of level III mosaicism for 47,XXY (46,XY/47,XXY), the presence of a significant fraction of chromosomally normal cells would be expected to moderate the expression of Klinefelter syndrome and the likelihood for near normal development is increased. However, important aspects of the expression of the symptoms of Klinefelter syndrome depend on the percentage and location of the cells with the extra X chromosome, e.g., brain and testes, information that is not available either prenatally or after birth, regardless of whether 47,XXY cells are recovered in a fetal blood sample.

Mosaicism for a 45,X cell line, either 45,X/46,XX or 45,X/46,XY, has a wide phenotypic spectrum. For 45,X/46,XX mosaicism, there is a phenotypic continuum ranging from the common findings of Turner syndrome to a normal or near normal female. Similarly, males with 45,X/46,XY mosaicism may have varying degrees of ambiguous genitalia or abnormal male genitalia of variable severity, structural abnormalities of the heart and kidneys seen in Turner syndrome, or have a normal or near normal male phenotype. Retrospective data collected about individuals diagnosed postnatally with 45,X/46,XY mosaicism include mainly those individuals who come to medical attention because of structural and/or functional abnormalities and thus cannot be used to provide prognostic information prospectively when the diagnosis of 45,X/46,XY mosaicism is made prenatally.

Predictions about adverse effects on development when 45,X/46,XY mosaicism is present in chorionic villi or amniocytes can be best made by detailed ultrasonographic examination. If fetal anatomy appears normal and the fetus has normally formed male genitalia, there is a high probability (>95%) of a normal-appearing baby at birth although there is a presumed increased risk of abnormal gonadal histology and germ cell tumors. Unfortunately, information about pubertal development, fertility, and risks of malignancy are not yet available for phenotypically normal boys who have been prenatally diagnosed with 45,X/46,XY mosaicism. Because of the possible increased risk of germ cell tumors in this group of boys, careful surveillance is indicated.

For prenatally diagnosed 45,X/46,XX mosaicism, if ultrasonographic examination shows absence of increased nuchal thickening, cystic hygroma, and heart and renal malformations, the risks of lymphatic abnormalities and other structural birth defects often seen in Turner syndrome will be small, but not eliminated. The risks of short stature and ovarian failure are increased but their degree cannot be predicted; there may be gonadal dysgenesis typical of Turner syndrome, less severe effects on ovarian function and fertility, or no apparent effects at all of the 45,X cell line.

In summary, when 45,X/46,XX and 45,X/46,XY mosaicism is detected in chorionic villi or amniotic fluid cells, the recovery of 45,X cells from a fetal tissue is unlikely to add information above that obtained from ultrasonographic examination. Mosaicism for a 45,X cell line can be explored after birth by chromosome studies of peripheral or cord blood cells, skin, including foreskin, or buccal mucosa.

Further reading

1 Bui TH, Iselius L, Lindsten J (1984) European collaborative study on prenatal diagnosis: mosaicism, pseudomosaicism and single abnormal cells in amniotic fluid cell cultures. *Prenatal Diagnosis* **4**:145–162.

2 Chang HJ, Clark RD, Bachman H (1990) The phenotype of 45,X/46,XY mosaicism: an analysis of 92 prenatally diagnosed cases. *American Journal of Human Genetics* **46**:156–167.

3 de Pater JM, Schuring-Blom GH, Nieste-Otter MA *et al.* (2000) Trisomy 8 in chorionic villi:

unpredictable results in follow-up. *Prenatal Diagnosis* **20**(5):435–437.

4 European Collaborative Research on Mosaicism in CVS (EUCROMIC) (1999) Trisomy 15 CPM: probable origins, pregnancy outcome and risk of fetal UPD. *Prenatal Diagnosis* **19**(1):29–35.

5 Hsu LYF, Perlis TE (1983) United States Survey on chromosome mosaicism and pseudomosaicism in prenatal diagnosis. *Prenatal Diagnosis* **4**:97–130.

6 Hsu LY, Yu MT, Neu RL *et al.* (1997) Rare trisomy mosaicism diagnosed in amniocytes, involving an autosome other than chromosomes 13, 18, 20, and 21: karyotype/phenotype correlations. *Prenatal Diagnosis* **17**(3):201–242.

7 Johnson A, Wapner RJ, Davis GH *et al.* (1990) Mosaicism in chorionic villus sampling: an association with poor perinatal outcome. *Obstetrics and Gynecology* **75**:573–577.

8 Kalousek DK, Howard-Peebles PN, Olson SB *et al.* (1991) Confirmation of CVS mosaicism in term placentae and high frequency of intrauterine growth retardation: association with confined placental mosaicism. *Prenatal Diagnosis* **11**:743–750.

9 Langlois S, Yong PJ, Yong SL *et al.* (2006) Postnatal follow-up of prenatally diagnosed trisomy 16 mosaicism. *Prenatal Diagnosis* **26**:548–558.

10 Ledbetter DH, Martin AO, Verlinsky Y *et al.* (1990) Cytogenetic results of chorionic villus sampling: high success rate and diagnostic accuracy in the United States collaborative study. *American Journal of Obstetrics and Gynecology* **162**:495–501.

11 Purvis-Smith SG, Saville T, Manass S *et al.* (1992) Uniparental disomy 15 resulting from "correction" of an initial trisomy 15. *American Journal of Human Genetics* **50**:1348–1350.

12 van Haelst MM, Van Opstal D, Lindhout D *et al.* (2001) Management of prenatally diagnosed trisomy 8 mosaicism. *Prenatal Diagnosis* **21**:1075–1078.

13 Vejerslev LO, Mikkelsen M (1989) The European collaborative study of mosaicism in chorionic villus sampling: data from 1986–1987. *Prenatal Diagnosis* **9**:575–588.

14 Worton RG, Stern R (1984) A Canadian collaborative study of mosaicism in amniotic fluid cell cultures. *Prenatal Diagnosis* **4**:131–144.

15 Yong PJ, Barrett IJ, Kalousek DK *et al.* (2003) Clinical aspects, prenatal diagnosis, and pathogenesis of trisomy 16 mosaicism. *Journal of Medical Genetics* **40**:175–182.

16 http://mosaicism.cfri.ca/index.htm

Chromosomal mosaicism – postnatal diagnosis

A 27-year-old woman and her husband are referred for genetic counseling because her peripheral blood karyotype obtained after the woman's second early miscarriage showed mosaicism for a 45,X cell line in 43% of her cells. The husband has a normal karyotype. The woman is 5'7' tall, has no external stigmata of Turner syndrome and has had normal renal and cardiac ultrasonographic examinations. She has a normal follicle stimulating hormone level.

Individuals with Turner syndrome mosaicism may have no signs of the syndrome, may have some manifestations of Turner syndrome, or may have all of the problems typically associated with non-mosaic Turner syndrome. The wide range of severity of findings in Turner syndrome mosaicism reflects the percentage and distribution of cells missing an X chromosome in various tissues. Individuals with Turner syndrome mosaicism who have functioning ovaries are at increased risk for premature ovarian failure. It is not possible to predict whether or when this might occur.

If the woman is able to conceive another pregnancy, she would be at increased risk for conceiving an embryo which is missing an X chromosome; almost all of these embryos would not survive beyond a few weeks' gestation. Thus, individuals with Turner syndrome mosaicism often have an increased risk of early pregnancy loss. There are conflicting data about whether she would also have an increased risk for conceptuses with other chromosomal abnormalities. If the woman can successfully conceive and carry a pregnancy through the end of the first trimester, there is a good chance of a normal outcome.

Prenatal diagnosis by chorionic villus sampling or amniocentesis could be performed to address the risk of chromosomal abnormalities. If the woman wishes to avoid an invasive procedure, first and second trimester serum screening and ultrasonography would also be reasonable approaches to provide information about the risk of common chromosomal abnormalities and other birth defects. Most fetuses with Turner syndrome would have visible stigmata on ultrasonographic examination.

Whether to recommend in vitro fertilization with preimplantation genetic diagnosis to increase the chance of implantation of a chromosomally normal embryo is unclear for this woman's situation. Her risk of fetal chromosomal abnormalities is unknown although the risk is probably increased over her age-related risks.

In the event that the woman experiences premature ovarian failure, pregnancy could be achieved via in vitro fertilization using an egg donated by another woman.

Further reading

1 Baena N, De Vigan C, Cariati E *et al.* (2003) Turner syndrome: evaluation of prenatal diagnosis in 19 European registries. *American Journal of Medical Genetics* **129A**(1):16–20.

2 Gunther DF, Eugster E, Zagar AJ *et al.* (2004) Ascertainment bias in Turner syndrome: new insights from girls who were diagnosed incidentally in prenatal life. *Pediatrics* **114**(3):640–644.

Sex discrepancies

Case 1 *A 38-year-old woman elects amniocentesis based on maternal age. First and second trimester aneuploidy screening had not been performed. The amniocyte karyotype was 46,XY and there was a normal amniotic fluid alpha-fetoprotein concentration. A follow-up ultrasonographic examination at 20 weeks' gestation revealed female-appearing genitalia.*

There are a number of explanations for a discrepancy between the chromosomal and phenotypic sex in this case.

• *Errors in ultrasonographic designation of the fetal sex.* At this gestational age, ultrasonographic anatomy is almost always correct in gender identification but circumstances such as ambiguous genitalia or micropenis and bifid scrotum might lead to the impression of female external genitalia when, in fact, some other conclusion would be made on direct visual examination.

• *Misidentified laboratory specimens.* Prevention of sample mix-ups should be of highest priority for any prenatal diagnosis program. Confirming proper sample labeling with the patient immediately following an invasive procedure and meticulous and redundant laboratory procedures are crucial components to preventing sample mix-ups. However, despite the most careful safeguards, occasional mistakes occur. Large studies of sample identification errors in clinical laboratory testing, indicate that the frequency of mislabeled samples ranges widely among different laboratories around the world.

• *Fetal pathology.* Fetal pathology must be considered as a possibility in this circumstance.

Another amniocentesis was recommended to confirm the chromosomal sex.

> *The karyotype of amniotic fluid cells obtained from the second amniocentesis was 46,XY, confirming the results of the first amniocentesis, allowing the possibility of a misidentified sample to be dismissed.*

In this situation there is discordance between the female external appearance of the fetus and the 46,XY karyotype, and the differential diagnosis includes several entities. These would include *SRY* mutations or deletions, androgen receptor mutations and other causes of androgen insensitivity, Smith–Lemli–Opitz syndrome, early errors in steroidogenesis, gonadal dysgenesis, several autosomal chromosome deletions or duplications, *SOX9* mutations that would usually show findings of campomelic dysplasia, Leydig cell hypoplasia, *DAX1* duplications at Xp21, true hermaphroditism, Denys–Drash syndrome, Wilms tumor syndromes, and others. Many of these are uncommon causes of the key findings and none of them makes up a large fraction of the differential.

Further diagnostic studies could include comparative genomic hybridization for chromosomal deletions and duplications and androgen receptor gene sequencing, which finds most autosomal recessive mutations in that gene. These molecular tests utilize DNA obtained from available cultured amniocytes, repeat amniocentesis, or placental biopsy. Measurement of 7-dehydrocholesterol, the abnormal metabolite diagnostic of Smith–Lemli–Opitz syndrome, could be performed on amniotic fluid supernatant. Further anatomic information might be possible with additional ultrasonographic examinations over subsequent weeks.

> *The patient had another detailed ultrasonographic examination and fetal echocardiography which revealed a complete atrioventricular canal defect and long bone measurements which lagged behind predicted gestational age.*

When the fetus is a chromosomal male, a discrepancy between the chromosomal and phenotypic sex, regardless of the presence or absence of other birth defects, should prompt strong consideration of Smith–Lemli–Opitz syndrome. Smith–Lemli–Opitz syndrome is an autosomal recessive disorder of cholesterol biosynthesis caused by a deficiency of 7-dehydrocholesterol reductase with an incidence in northern Europeans as high as 1 in 10 000. It is characterized by prenatal and postnatal growth retardation, ambiguous genitalia in males, microcephaly, moderate to severe mental retardation, and multiple major and minor malformations. Affected individuals have markedly elevated levels of 7-dehydrocholesterol and may have hypocholesterolemia. The prenatal diagnosis of Smith–Lemli–Opitz syndrome is accomplished by measurement of 7-dehydrocholesterol in amniotic fluid supernatant or chorionic villus cells.

> *In this patient's pregnancy, 7-dehydrocholesterol was assayed in frozen amniotic fluid supernatant from both amniocenteses and was markedly elevated, confirming the diagnosis of Smith–Lemli–Opitz syndrome. Establishing a definitive diagnosis allowed for the provision of accurate information about prognosis, risk of recurrence, and the availability of early prenatal diagnosis in future pregnancies by measurement of 7-dehydrocholesterol in chorionic villus cells. Mutations in only one gene, DHCR7, are known to cause Smith–Lemli–Opitz syndrome. If the disease-causing mutation(s) are identified in this conception, preimplantation genetic diagnosis and DNA-based diagnosis using chorionic villus or amniotic fluid cells would also be possible in future pregnancies.*

Case 2 A 41-year-old primiparous woman elected chorionic villus sampling at 11 weeks' gestation. The karyotype from cultured chorionic villus cells was 46,XX. Detailed ultrasonographic examination was performed at 18 weeks' gestation and revealed normal appearing fetal anatomy. The fetal genitalia appeared male and this was confirmed on a subsequent ultrasonogram.

There are a number of explanations for a discrepancy between the chromosomal and phenotypic sex in this case.

• *Errors in ultrasonographic designation of the fetal sex.* At this gestational age, ultrasonographic anatomy is almost always correct in gender identification.

• *Misidentified laboratory specimens.* Despite the most careful safeguards, sample error can still occur at the time of the procedure or in the laboratory, as discussed in the previous case of XY genotype and female phenotype.

• *Maternal cell contamination.* Unrecognized maternal cell contamination is a negligible concern when villi are expertly dissected and harvested for cytogenetic analysis after a few days in culture.

• *Fetal pathology.* Fetal pathology must be considered as a possibility in this circumstance.

Amniocentesis was recommended to confirm the chromosomal sex.

The karyotype of amniotic fluid cells obtained from amniotic fluid cells was 46,XX, confirming the results of chorionic villus sampling, dismissing the possibility of a misidentified laboratory specimen as an explanation.

The most likely explanations for the discrepancy between the fetal karyotype and phenotype include: (1) a male fetus with the *SRY* gene that encodes the testis-determining factor. This may result from a translocation between the *SRY* gene from a Y chromosome and the pseudoautosomal region of the X chromosome, or translocation between the *SRY* gene and an autosome; and (2) a female fetus with excessive androgen synthesis due to an enzyme deficiency in the pathways of steroidogenesis. These enzyme deficiencies all have autosomal recessive inheritance. The most common is 21-hydroxylase deficiency which has a high incidence in Ashkenazi Jews and is caused by mutations in the *CYP21A2* gene. In 46,XX females of any ethnic group, genetic disorders associated with excessive androgen production are a common cause of virilization. In contrast, in 46,XY males, abnormalities in the androgen synthesis pathway are a rare cause of sexual ambiguity.

Further diagnostic studies could include fluorescence in situ hybridization (FISH) analysis of DNA from cultured amniocytes to look for the presence of the *SRY* gene. Results of FISH analysis are usually available within one to two days.

If FISH analysis of DNA obtained from amniotic fluid cells were negative for the *SRY* gene, mutation analysis of the parents' 21-hydroylase genes could be undertaken. Mutation analysis has a greater than 95% sensitivity in the detection of disease-causing mutations but may take several weeks to accomplish. If both parents have identifiable mutations, the a priori risk of 21-hydroxylase deficiency in the fetus would be 25% and definitive testing of DNA obtained from cultured amniocytes to confirm 21-hydroxylase deficiency as the explanation of the virilized fetus could be accomplished. If neither or only one parent has an identifiable mutation in their 21-hydroxylase gene, the chance that 21-hydroxylase deficiency is the explanation for the fetal problems would be small.

There are major limitations to prenatal diagnosis of other disorders of steroidogenesis that could result in a virilized female fetus. Other genes coding for steroidogenic enzymes not involved in androgen biosynthesis, such as P450aro, must also be considered, as mutations in these can result in overproduction of androgens, resulting in disorders of sex determination. All are rare conditions. Enzyme testing of amniotic fluid is not available because these enzymes are not expressed in amniotic fluid cells or present in amniotic fluid supernatant. Unfortunately, mutation testing of known genes is not likely to be practical.

In this patient's pregnancy, FISH analysis of amniotic fluid cells identified the presence of the SRY gene, the sex-determining region of the Y chromosome. This occurred presumably due to an abnormal X-Y or Y-autosome interchange during spermatogenesis in the patient's husband who has a normal (46,XY) karyotype. He has three children (two daughters and one son) from a previous marriage. The X-Y or Y-autosome interchange arose as a de novo event in the pregnancy and has a low risk of recurrence in future conceptions.

Further reading

1 College of American Pathologists, Valenstein PN, Raab SS *et al.* (2006) Identification errors involving clinical laboratories: a College of American Pathologists Q-Probes study of patient and specimen identification errors at 120 institutions. *Archives of Pathology and Laboratory Medicine* **130**(8):1106–1113.

2 Cost NG, Ludwig AT, Wilcox DT *et al.* (2009) A novel SOX9 mutation, 972delC, causes 46,XY sex-reversed campomelic dysplasia with nephrocalcinosis, urolithiasis, and dysgerminoma. *Journal of Pediatric Surgery* **44**(2):451–454.

3 Dzik WH, Murphy MF, Andreu G *et al.* (2003) An international study of the performance of sample collection from patients. *Vox Sanguinis* **85**:40–47.

4 Ergun-Longmire B, Vinci G, Alonso L *et al.* (2005) Clinical, hormonal and cytogenetic evaluation of 46,XX males and review of the literature. *Journal of Pediatric Endocrinology and Metabolism* **18**(8):739–748.

5 Ginsberg NA, Cadkin A, Strom C *et al.* (1999) Prenatal diagnosis of 46,XX male fetuses. *American Journal of Obstetrics and Gynecology* **180**(4):1006–1007.

6 MacLaughlin DT, Donahoe PK (2004) Sex determination and differentiation. *New England Journal of Medicine* **350**:367–378.

7 McElreavey K, Barbaux S, Ion A *et al.* (1995) The genetic basis of murine and human sex determination: a review. *Heredity* **75**(Pt 6):599–611.

8 Mendonca BB, Domenice S, Arnhold IJ *et al.* (2009) 46,XY disorders of sex development (DSD). *Clinical Endocrinology* **70**:173–187.

9 Odeh M, Granin V, Kais M *et al.* (2009) Sonographic fetal sex determination. *Obstetrics and Gynecology Survey* **64**(1):50–57.

10 Pajkrt E, Petersen OB, Chitty LS. (2008) Fetal genital anomalies: an aid to diagnosis. *Prenatal Diagnosis* 28 (5):389–98.

11 Pinhas-Hamiel O, Zalel Y, Smith E *et al.* (2002) Prenatal diagnosis of sex differentiation disorders: the role of fetal ultrasound. ***Journal of Clinical Endocrinology and Metabolism*** **87**(10): 4547–4553.

12 Sarafoglou K, Ostrer H (2000) Clinical Review 111: Familial sex reversal: a review. *Journal of Clinical Endocrinology and Metabolism* **85**(2): 483–493.

2 Mendelian Inheritance

Prenatal Diagnosis: Cases & Clinical Challenges, 1st edition. By Miriam S. DiMaio, Joyce E. Fox, Maurice J. Mahoney
Published 2010 by Blackwell Publishing Ltd.

Introduction to Mendelian inheritance

Disorders with Mendelian inheritance, which are also known as single gene disorders, are due to major effects of one or both members of a pair of genes. The separation of these genes during meiosis with each ovum or sperm receiving only one copy of that gene is known as Mendel's Law of Segregation. Thus, the genes which cause Mendelian disorders are transmitted in a predictable pattern from one generation to the next. There are rare circumstances in which single gene disorders can arise in violation of Mendelian inheritance. Uniparental disomy in which both copies of a gene are transmitted from one parent is one example. However, Mendelian inheritance still applies for the vast majority of families in which a single gene disorder is present.

Hundreds of Mendelian disorders are amenable to prenatal diagnosis by molecular analysis. Counseling about the results of prenatal diagnostic testing for these conditions is usually straightforward when the disorder is consistently associated with a narrow range of clinical abnormalities, the diagnosis of the affected family members has been clearly established, or the nucleotide change(s) that have been identified in a gene are already known to be pathogenic. Such an example is Tay–Sachs disease, where homozygosity or compound heterozygosity for common mutations in the *HEXA* gene invariably results in a fatal neurodegenerative course during the first years of life.

However, such ideal counseling situations are often not the reality. For some disorders, such as X-linked adrenoleukodystrophy, a devastating neurodegenerative course during the first decade of life may affect one family member while, in another, milder neurologic impairment develops only in adulthood. Such a wide spectrum in severity and age of onset of symptoms among family members who have the same mutation are also the hallmarks of many autosomal dominant disorders, as illustrated by tuberous sclerosis. Phenotypic heterogeneity can also be seen in autosomal recessive disorders such as spinal muscular atrophy in which known and unknown genetic modifiers influence severity of disease. Although prenatal diagnosis of a disorder is highly accurate once a disease causing mutation(s) has been identified in a family, precise predictions about expression of the phenotype are sometimes not possible to make and complicate decision making about whether to pursue prenatal diagnosis or consider pregnancy termination.

For some disorders, counseling is complicated by the identification of a novel nucleotide change of uncertain pathologic significance in an affected family member. Establishing the pathogenicity of such an unreported nucleotide change may not be possible, thus leaving doubt about the accuracy of preimplantation or prenatal genetic diagnosis.

Another obstacle to providing accurate risk estimates is the phenomenon of genetic heterogeneity where mutations in more than one gene can lead to the same or similar phenotype. At times, there may even be a different mode of inheritance. Incorrect assumptions about an inheritance pattern can lead to erroneous assessments of risk in a fetus and missed opportunities for prenatal diagnosis. If confirmatory clinical and/or diagnostic laboratory testing has not been accomplished for an affected relative, the estimation of risk to a fetus must be made cautiously.

These challenges and basic concepts related to single gene inheritance including pedigree interpretation, calculation of risk estimates, the Hardy–Weinberg equilibrium, atypical X-linked inheritance, factors influencing expression of an X-linked disease in females, and trinucleotide repeat expansions are presented here.

Autosomal dominant disorders

Features of autosomal dominant inheritance

1 The trait (phenotype) appears if the abnormal gene is present on only one homologous autosomal chromosome.

2 Each child of an affected individual has a 50% chance of inheriting the gene.

3 Males and females are affected with equal frequency and transmit the abnormal gene to sons and daughters with equal frequency.

4 Family members who do not carry the abnormal gene do not transmit the trait to their children.

5 There can be a wide range in the severity and age of onset of the trait (variable expression).

6 For some autosomal dominant disorders, a percentage of individuals with the abnormal gene do not express the trait although they can transmit it, which then gives the appearance of "skipped" generations (incomplete penetrance).

Autosomal dominant polycystic kidney disease

A couple comes for genetic counseling because the 31-year-old husband reports that he has polycystic kidney disease diagnosed by renal imaging performed as a teenager after his father developed end-stage renal disease at age 40 years due to polycystic kidney disease. His father and paternal grandfather died of a stroke in their early 40s. It is not known whether the paternal grandfather had polycystic kidney disease. The husband is an only child, as was his father. The husband's mother is alive at age 78 years. The husband reports that he has hypertension, which is well controlled by antihypertensive medications, and that he has regular brain imaging by MRI. The couple wants to avoid the birth of a child who will develop polycystic kidney disease.

Autosomal dominant polycystic kidney disease (ADPKD) is one of the most common single gene disorders, affecting about 1 in 800 individuals. The disorder, which usually begins in mid-life, often has extrarenal manifestations which include cysts in the liver, pancreas, and seminal vesicles. In addition, there is an increased risk of intracranial aneurysm, stroke and dissection of the thoracic aorta due to weakening of the arterial wall.

Mutations in two genes, *PKD1* and *PKD2*, account for 85% and 15% of cases, respectively. Mutations in other gene(s) may cause disease in rare families in whom no identifiable mutation in *PKD1* or *PKD2* can be detected and no linkage to either of these genes can be established.

The variable expression and pleiotropic effects of the disorder can in part be explained by the underlying molecular pathogenesis, as well as other, yet unidentified, genetic and environmental factors. Compared with *PKD2* gene mutations, *PKD1* gene mutations are associated with more severe disease expression including earlier age of onset, an increased chance of associated complications, earlier onset of end-stage renal failure, and earlier age at death. For example, almost all carriers of a *PKD1* gene mutation, but only two-thirds of *PKD2* gene mutation carriers, will have renal cysts evident on ultrasonographic examination by age 30 years.

Gene sequencing and duplication-deletion testing of *PKD1* and *PKD2* are available through clinical diagnostic laboratories.

The husband submits a blood sample for molecular testing of his PKD1 *and* PKD2 *genes. No pathogenic nucleotide changes were found in his* PKD2 *genes. Analysis of his* PKD1 *genes identified a nucleotide change involving a transversion from guanine to cytosine at codon 2266. The laboratory report states that this finding could be either a benign polymorphism or a disease-associated mutation, but did not provide further information.*

A number of criteria can be used to help distinguish a pathogenic mutation from a silent, benign polymorphism. These include the following:

1 The nucleotide change has been reported in other families with ADPKD by searching the Polycystic Kidney Disease Mutation Database which is accessible by internet and updated frequently.

2 The nucleotide change segregates with PKD in the family. Do all affected family members have the nucleotide change while unaffected family members do not?

3 The nucleotide change is predicted to cause a significant alteration in the protein structure. Major changes in the structure of the protein are often associated with abnormalities of function.

4 The normal DNA sequence has remained the same among different mammalian and other species, suggesting, in evolutionary conservation terms, that it is very important for normal functioning.

Review of the Polycystic Kidney Disease Mutation Database showed that the nucleotide change in the husband has not been reported in other affected individuals. Demonstrating segregation of the nucleotide change with ADPKD in the husband's family is not possible as there are no other living affected family members.

However, two lines of evidence give fairly strong support that the nucleotide change found in the husband is a disease-associated mutation. First, the DNA alteration is predicted to substantially alter the protein product of the gene based on modeling programs by biochemists. Second, the normal DNA sequence at codon 2266 in the PKD1 gene is highly conserved among different mammalian species and among fish.

Whether the couple should proceed with preimplantation or prenatal genetic diagnosis for ADPKD based on the available information suggesting that the nucleotide change is pathogenic requires careful consideration. The evidence for pathogenicity is good but not definitive. Before proceeding with a pregnancy, testing of the husband's unaffected mother to determine whether she has the nucleotide change or normal gene sequence would provide some additional information. If she has the nucleotide change present in her son, this would be strong evidence that it is not disease-causing. Absence of the nucleotide change in the mother would show that it was transmitted from his affected father, barring new mutation or non-paternity, and provides evidence of segregation of the nucleotide change with disease status. To prove in a statistically meaningful way that a nucleotide variant segregates with disease status, many affected and unaffected individuals in a family would need to be studied, something that is not possible given the very small size of the husband's family.

The husband's mother has DNA testing which shows that she does not carry the PKD1 gene nucleotide change identified in her son.

Information about the mother provides further support for the pathogenicity of the nucleotide change. Unfortunately, no further testing is currently available that can provide definitive information for this family. As more information is gathered into DNA databases about ADPKD families, it is possible that other families will be reported with a similar gene alteration. This information may not be forthcoming for several years, and the couple will need to make reproductive decisions with less than perfect information.

Further reading

1 Brun M, Maugey-Laulom B, Eurin D *et al.* (2004) Prenatal sonographic patterns in autosomal dominant polycystic kidney disease: a multicenter study. *Ultrasound in Obstetrics and Gynecology* 24:55–61.

2 Harris PC, Torres VE (Updated 6/2/2009) Polycystic Kidney Disease, Autosomal Dominant. In: *GeneReviews* at GeneTests: Medical Genetics Information Resource (database online). Copyright, University of Washington, Seattle. 1997–2009. Available at http://www.genetests.org. Accessed September 2009.

3 Pei Y (2003) Molecular genetics of autosomal dominant polycystic kidney disease. *Clinical and Investigative Medicine* 26(5):252–258.

4 Vora N, Perrone R, Bianchi DW (2008) Reproductive issues for adults with autosomal dominant polycystic kidney disease. *American Journal of Kidney Disease* 51(2):307–318.

5 Wilson PD (2004) Polycystic kidney disease. *New England Journal of Medicine* 350:151–164.

Hereditary colon cancer

A 25-year-old man is newly married and comes for genetic counseling with his wife to learn about reproductive options. The man has known for several years that he carries a mutation in one of his MLH1 genes, one of the genes associated with hereditary non-polyposis colon cancer (HNPCC). He had testing as a teenager at the urging of his mother who was diagnosed with colon cancer at age 30 years. The man's family history also includes a maternal aunt, maternal grandmother and maternal great grandfather who were all diagnosed with colon cancer in their 30s. The man has yearly colonoscopies.

Mutations in the *MLH1* gene, one of the genes involved in DNA mismatch repair, are associated with an increased risk of HNPCC. Individuals who carry a DNA mismatch repair mutation have a lifetime risk of developing HNPCC of about 80% as well as increased risk of other cancers including cancers of the endometrium, ovary, stomach, small intestine, hepatobiliary tract, upper urinary tract, brain, and skin. HNPCC has autosomal dominant inheritance. Five percent of all cases of colon cancer are due to HNPCC.

Each of the couple's children has a 50% risk of inheriting his *MLH1* gene mutation and a high lifetime risk of cancer. If the couple wants to avoid the birth of a child with the *MLH1* gene mutation, preimplantation genetic diagnosis could be utilized to select for embryos which are unaffected. Prenatal diagnosis by chorionic villus sampling or amniocentesis could also be performed although most couples are not inclined to consider pregnancy termination for conditions that usually do not have manifestations until mid-life. Another alternative would be artificial insemination with sperm from an unrelated donor or an unaffected male relative of the husband. If the sperm donor is related to the husband, he should be screened for the familial *MLH1* gene mutation. An unrelated sperm donor could also be screened for an *MLH1* gene mutation although the chance of such a donor having that mutation would be extremely low, and the *MLH1* gene is only one of many genes whose mutations carry a high lifetime cancer risk.

The couple states that they are being strongly encouraged to have preimplantation genetic diagnosis by the husband's family to eliminate the risk of HNPCC in future generations. They, however, state that they are much more inclined to conceive a child naturally and hope that better therapies for cancer prevention are developed by the time their children reach adulthood.

Further reading

1 Kastrinos F, Stoffel EM, Balmana J *et al.* (2007) Attitudes toward prenatal genetic testing in patients with familial adenomatous polyposis. *American Journal of Gastroenterology* **102**(6):1284–1290.
2 Spits C, DeRycke M, Van Ranst N *et al.* (2007) Preimplantation genetic diagnosis for cancer pre-disposition syndromes. *Prenatal Diagnosis* **27**(5):447–456.
3 Tops CM, Wijnen JT, Hes FJ (2009) Introduction to molecular and clinical genetics of colorectal cancer syndromes. *Best Practices and Research, Clinical Gastroenterology* **23**(2):127–146.

Huntington disease

A woman is referred for genetic counseling in the first trimester because the family history collected by her obstetrician includes relatives of her husband who reportedly have Huntington disease. His mother, maternal grandmother, two maternal aunts, and a female maternal first cousin have the disorder or have died from its complications. The husband states that his mother died at age 58 years after a 20-year course of the disease. Two maternal uncles are in their 60s and unaffected. The husband is 38

years old and in good health. He has two brothers who are reported to be well in their 30s.

Huntington disease is an autosomal dominant neurodegenerative disorder usually characterized by progressively worsening involuntary movements, cognitive impairment, and psychiatric disturbance. There is a wide range in age of onset from early childhood to old age, although the majority of affected individuals develop symptoms between ages 30 and 50 years. The molecular basis of Huntington disease is a trinucleotide repeat expansion in one copy of the *huntingtin* gene in which the number of CAG repeats that exceed a certain threshold will eventually result in manifestations of the disorder. Age of onset of symptoms is correlated with the size of the CAG expansion. Alleles with CAG expansions are unstable during male meiosis, resulting in the phenomenon of anticipation in which the offspring of affected males often have an earlier onset of symptoms due to large trinucleotide expansions in one of their Huntington disease genes.

Because other neurodegenerative disorders can occasionally mimic the symptoms of Huntington disease, it is important to confirm that at least one affected member of the family has had the clinical diagnosis confirmed by molecular testing to provide the most accurate genetic counseling, especially if the husband would be considering molecular testing of his own Huntington disease genes. If Huntington disease is the correct diagnosis for the husband's relatives, he has a 50% chance of having inherited his mother's abnormal Huntington disease gene and developing symptoms of the disorder at some point in his life.

A review of the affected maternal cousin's molecular testing shows that she has one normal-sized Huntington disease gene and another allele with 42 CAG repeats (normal range < 36 CAG repeats). This result confirms the clinical diagnosis of Huntington disease in the husband's family.

The couple is surprised to learn that the husband is at risk for developing Huntington disease. Because no males in his family are known to have the disorder, he and his relatives were under the strong impression that males were not susceptible.

The distortion in the sex distribution of individuals affected with autosomal dominant conditions is not uncommon in small families and is almost always due to chance. The husband's family is an example of how such distortions in the sex ratio of affected relatives often lead to misinformation and mythologies in these families about who is actually at risk for developing the disorder.

When a parent of either sex carries an autosomal dominant mutation, each of his or her children, regardless of sex, has a 50% chance of inheriting that mutant gene. When a large number of families with Huntington disease (or other autosomal dominant disorders) is studied, there is an equal sex distribution of affected individuals.

The husband has a 50% chance of having inherited his mother's mutant Huntington disease gene.

Both the woman and her husband cared for his mother during her illness and are familiar with the course of the disorder. The woman is now concerned about her husband's Huntington disease gene status and the possibility that he also will develop symptoms of the disorder. She also wants prenatal testing of the fetal Huntington disease genes although she doubts that pregnancy termination is a consideration. The husband is unsure about whether he wants to learn about his own Huntington disease gene status.

For the husband, due to the current pregnancy, this is an extremely difficult time to learn that he is at 50% risk for a neurodegenerative disorder and may have already transmitted an abnormal gene for that disorder to a child. Whether to have presymptomatic testing for a disorder which currently does not have any effective treatment or prevention requires careful consideration. Abnormal results of such testing may have significant ramifications for psychological well-being and may influence professional, vocational and educational goals, financial planning, and reproductive decisions. Genetic counseling with professionals experienced in this area is strongly recommended.

If prenatal testing by chorionic villus sampling or amniocentesis is undertaken, fetal testing which reveals that the fetus has an abnormal Huntington disease gene will be diagnostic of the husband's Huntington disease gene status, information that he may not want. In addition, fetal testing is tantamount to testing a child for a condition that usually does not manifest symptoms until adult life and for which there is no current therapy which can prevent or delay onset of symptoms. Professional guidelines strongly discourage testing of minors for such adult-onset conditions. The consensus of these guidelines is that it is preferable to let individuals make autonomous decisions as adults about whether they want this information or not, and that it is preferable to avoid the situation where children might be treated differently by their parents or others if they are known to carry an

abnormal gene, even if that gene is unlikely to cause problems for several decades.

The scenario described above raises difficult ethical and legal issues that involve the right of the woman to have information about her fetus, the right of the husband to avoid learning his Huntington disease gene status if he prefers not to know, and the right of the child to make his or her own decision about whether and when to learn of his or her Huntington disease gene status.

For a future pregnancy if the husband does not wish to learn of his Huntington disease gene status but wants to avoid the birth of a child with the abnormal Huntington disease gene, in vitro fertilization with non-disclosing preimplantation genetic diagnosis could be performed. In this scenario, only embryos that are shown to have two normal Huntington disease genes would be implanted in the wife's womb or frozen for future use, but the couple would not be informed as to whether any abnormal embryos were found.

Further reading

1 Brinkman RR Mezei MM, Theilmann J *et al.* (1997) The likelihood of being affected with Huntington disease by a particular age, for a specific CAG size. *American Journal of Human Genetics* **60**(5):1202–1210.
2 Stevanin G, Fujigasaki H, Lebre AS *et al.* (2003) Huntington's disease-like phenotype due to trinucleotide repeat expansions in the TBP and JPH3 genes. *Brain* **126**:1599–1603.
3 Tassicker R, Savulescu J, Skene L *et al.* (2003) Prenatal diagnosis requests for Huntington's disease when the father is at risk and does not want to know his genetic status: clinical, legal, and ethical viewpoints. *British Medical Journal* **326**:331–333.

Marfan syndrome

A 23-year-old woman is referred for genetic counseling at 13 weeks' gestation due to an increased risk for Down syndrome predicted by first trimester screening. Her family history includes her oldest son who reportedly had hypoplastic left heart syndrome and died at 3 months of age. The woman also reports that her mother, age 58 years, and her maternal grandfather were diagnosed with Marfan syndrome. Both are described as being about 6 feet tall with long arms and legs. Her grandfather died of a ruptured thoracic aortic aneurysm in his 50s. Her mother had repair of a thoracic aortic aneurysm a few years ago. A maternal uncle died of a stroke in his 50s. A maternal cousin died suddenly in his 30s of an unknown cause. The woman believes that she might have been evaluated for Marfan syndrome as a teenager and was not thought to have the disorder.

Because the woman could be affected by Marfan syndrome or another thoracic aortic aneurysm syndrome, echocardiography should be accomplished immediately with particular attention to her aortic root and to her aortic valve. In women with Marfan syndrome who have pre-existing aortic or mitral valve disease or dilatation of the aortic root, the hemodynamic changes during pregnancy significantly increase the risk of aortic dissection and death.

The woman's echocardiogram is normal and shows only minimal mitral valve prolapse. She was unaware that she could still have Marfan syndrome and have an affected child.

Although Marfan syndrome is a very possible diagnosis in the woman's mother, given the clinical presentations of the two people who have been labeled with that diagnosis and their dissecting aneurysms, there are other possible diagnoses. Thoracic aortic aneurysm syndromes are inherited in an autosomal dominant manner and some show cystic medial necrosis of the aortic wall, as does Marfan syndrome. Also, at times these aneurysms occur in families where there are aortic valve abnormalities and, rarely, hypoplastic left heart syndrome.

Marfan syndrome, an autosomal dominant disorder of connective tissue, has a wide range of clinical severity and is due to mutations in the *FBN1* (fibrillin) gene. Affected organ systems include the eye (myopia and lens dislocation), skeleton (bone overgrowth, scoliosis, and joint laxity), and heart (dilatation of the aorta root, predisposition for aortic dissection, mitral valve prolapse, triscuspid valve prolapse, and enlargement of the proximal pulmonary artery). Some individuals with mild presentations may not be recognized while the severe form can result in early death. The diagnosis is made using clinical criteria and family history. Mutations in the *FBN1* gene are also associated with other disorders which have clinical overlap with Marfan syndrome including the MASS phenotype (**m**yopia, **m**itral valve prolapse, **a**ortic enlargement, and non-specific **s**kin and **s**keletal features), mitral valve prolapse syndrome, and familial ectopia lentis. In addition, another group of disorders which are not associated with mutations in the *FBN1* gene also have clinical similarities to Marfan syndrome. These include

familial thoracic aortic aneurysms and aortic dissection (TAAD), vascular (type 4) Ehlers–Danlos syndrome, Loeys–Dietz syndrome, homocystinuria, and others.

Since the woman wants information about her own Marfan syndrome status and risks to her children, an evaluation by a medical geneticist is indicated to see whether her clinical presentation meets the diagnostic criteria for Marfan syndrome. If it does, then sequencing of her *FBN1* gene could be performed to look for a disease-causing mutation. Between 70–90% of *FBN1* gene mutations are identifiable by gene testing.

The woman has a genetics and ophthalmologic evaluation which does not support the diagnosis of Marfan syndrome.

It is not appropriate to initiate gene sequencing of the woman's *FBN1* genes as her clinical presentation does not meet the diagnostic criteria for Marfan syndrome. Identification of an *FBN1* gene mutation in the woman's mother (presuming that the mother has been correctly diagnosed with Marfan syndrome) would allow definitive exclusion of the woman's Marfan syndrome status. Clinical evaluation of the mother is warranted as she was diagnosed with Marfan syndrome many years ago, prior to the development of the criteria used to establish a firm clinical diagnosis of the disorder.

The woman's mother is evaluated by a medical geneticist and does not meet the clinical criteria for Marfan syndrome. However, the family history is strongly suggestive that the thoracic aortic aneurysms have an autosomal dominant basis.

In contrast to Marfan syndrome in which all cases are due to mutations in the *FBN1* gene, thoracic aneurysms (ascending and descending) associated with autosomal dominant inheritance show genetic heterogeneity. Also, in contrast to Marfan syndrome where mutations in the *FBN1* gene are usually completely penetrant (i.e., almost all carries of an *FBN1* gene mutation have manifestations of the disorder), there are families with autosomal dominant inheritance of thoracic aneurysms in which there are unaffected obligate carriers of a gene mutation. In some families, cerebral aneurysms are also present.

Mutations in four genes have been identified to cause thoracic aneurysms. However, sequence analysis of these genes identifies less than 20% of disease-causing mutations. Some families with thoracic aneurysms show linkage to other loci with as yet uncharacterized genes.

Whether the hypoplastic left heart syndrome in the woman's son was related to thoracic aneurysms affecting other family members is not known and cannot be established. It increases the probability that she is a carrier of a gene which causes thoracic aneurysms. Whether she will develop a thoracic aneurysm (or aneurysms elsewhere) in the future is not known. She should have surveillance for both thoracic and cerebral aneurysms, given the history of a cousin who died of a stroke at a young age. Because she has had a child with hypoplastic left heart syndrome, the risk of another child with congenital heart disease is at least a few percent. Fetal echocardiography is recommended in her pregnancy.

Further reading

1 Caglayan AO, Dundar M (2009) Inherited diseases and syndromes leading to aortic aneurysms and dissections. *European Journal of Cardiothoracic Surgery* **35**(6):931–940.

2 Dean JC (2007) Marfan syndrome: clinical diagnosis and management. *European Journal of Human Genetics* **15**(7):724–733.

3 Dietz H (updated 6/30/2009) Marfan Syndrome. In: *GeneReviews* at GeneTests: Medical Genetics Information Resource (database online). Copyright, University of Washington, Seattle. 1997–2009. Available at http://www.genetests.org. Accessed September 2009.

4 Krischek B, Inoue I (2006) The genetics of intracranial aneurysms. *Journal of Human Genetics* **51**(7):587–594.

5 Milewicz DM, Guo DC, Tran-Fadulu V *et al.* (2008) Genetic basis of thoracic aortic aneurysms and dissections: focus on smooth muscle cell contractile dysfunction. *Annual Review of Genomics and Human Genetics* **9**:283–302.

6 Pannu H, Tran-Fadulu V, Milewicz DM (2005) Genetic basis of thoracic aortic aneurysms and aortic dissections. *American Journal of Medical Genetics Part C: Seminars in Medical Genetics* **139C**1):10–16.

Retinoblastoma

A 28-year-old primiparous woman at 10 weeks' gestation is referred for genetic counseling because she was diagnosed with an advanced unilateral retinoblastoma at age 3 years in another country. At the time of diagnosis, she had metastases in her abdomen. She was treated with radiation and chemotherapy. After enucleation of her eye and completion of her treatment, she experienced no other medical problems. Her family history does not include other relatives with retinoblastoma.

This woman's history raises three important questions. The first is whether there might be consequences to the fetus from her prior treatment with chemotherapy and radiation. The second is whether there is a hereditary component to her retinoblastoma placing her children at increased risk of recurrence and susceptibility to other malignancies. The third is whether she faces other health consequences based on her having had a retinoblastoma.

Retinoblastoma is a rare childhood cancer. It may arise de novo in an individual or may be the consequence of an inherited mutation. Retinoblastoma is the paradigmatic disorder illustrating the phenomenon of the two-hit model of tumorigenesis.

Retinoblastoma arises when there is homozygosity for an inactivating mutation in the *RB1* gene, which is a tumor suppressor gene on the long arm of chromosome 13. One *RB1* gene mutation can be inherited from a parent or can arise de novo in a retinoblast during embryogenesis. A heterozygous inactivating mutation in a single *RB1* gene in a retinoblast is not sufficient to cause disease; however, it is a prerequisite for disease occurrence. The development of a retinoblastoma requires a "second hit," a mutation in the homologous *RB1* gene, on the other chromosome 13, which occurs as a result of a somatic mutation.

When *both* the "first hit" and "second hit" in the *RB1* gene arise as somatic events in the same retinoblast, the result is a unilateral retinoblastoma. In this case, the individual does not have an increased risk of recurrent retinoblastoma or other malignancies. On the other hand, if the "first hit" in the *RB1* gene is due to a germline mutation that has been inherited from a parent, there is an increased risk of multifocal tumors in the same eye, bilateral retinoblastoma due to "second hits" in both eyes and other non-ocular cancers due to "second hits" in the cells of other body tissues. The risk of cancer in other body tissues is correlated with the amount of radiation exposure with heavily irradiated sites having a higher risk, reflecting the higher chance of a radiation-induced "second hit." Inherited *RB1* mutations follow an autosomal dominant pattern of inheritance and cause what is known as the *RB1* cancer syndrome.

The woman's history does not allow us to establish whether she has a sporadic case of retinoblastoma or whether she has a germline mutation and is at risk for transmitting an *RB1* gene mutation to her children. In about 15% of individuals with unilateral retinoblastoma who have no family history of the disorder, one of the *RB1* gene mutations found in the tumor is also found in DNA obtained from the individual's peripheral blood. The mutation in the blood cells could be of germline origin inherited from a parent, or present in a mosaic state, having occurred as a somatic mutation after conception.

A pathologic specimen from the woman's tumor is not available. Sequencing of her RB1 genes is accomplished using DNA obtained from her peripheral blood cells. She is heterozygous for a previously described nucleotide change. DNA testing of her parents does not identify the RB1 gene mutation and examinations of their retinas are normal. The RB1 gene mutation arose due to a new mutation in either the ovum or sperm with which she was conceived, or might have occurred as a somatic mutation early in embryogenesis.

Each of this woman's children has a 50% chance of inheriting her *RB1* gene mutation. Of those with the mutation, 95% will develop a retinoblastoma in at least one eye, and all face a high lifetime risk of developing other cancers. These children need early surveillance by retinoblastoma specialists in ophthalmology and oncology. This woman could also have prenatal diagnosis of the *RB1* gene mutation or preimplantation genetic diagnosis for a future pregnancy. For a fetus who is at high risk or known to carry a *RB1* gene mutation, ultrasound surveillance is indicated. Some cases of retinoblastoma present during fetal life.

Gonadal function is adversely affected by prior radiation and chemotherapy resulting in increased risks of infertility or decreased fertility of varying degrees depending on the age of treatment, the type and dose of chemotherapy, and whether the pelvis and abdomen were irradiated. For women who become pregnant, the risk of spontaneous abortion is increased, especially among women previously exposed to high-dose radiation.

For women treated in childhood for non-hereditary cancers who are able to become pregnant, the available data indicate the risk of birth defects or childhood cancers in their children does not appear to be increased over that of the general population background risk. These data reflect the experience with older therapeutic agents and may not apply to the effects of newer treatment regimens available today, which include mutagenic drugs other than alkylating agents and may have different mutagenic effects. There are increased risks of prematurity and low birth weight for the offspring of childhood cancer survivors, with the risk primarily among women who have a history of abdominal radiation. This increased risk reflects radiation-induced damage to the uterus.

Because this woman has a significantly increased risk of second malignancies due to her germline *RB1* gene muta-

tion, particularly because she was irradiated, careful surveillance for second cancers is indicated. Avoidance of DNA-damaging agents such as tobacco and ultraviolet light may diminish the risk of some *RB1*-associated cancers.

Further reading

1 Boice JD Jr, Tawn EJ, Winther JF *et al.* (2003) Genetic effects of radiotherapy for childhood cancer. *Health Physics* **85**(1):65–80.

2 Green DM, Sklar CA, Boice JD *et al.* (2009) Ovarian failure and reproductive outcomes after childhood cancer treatment: results from the Childhood Cancer Survivor Study. *Journal of Clinical Oncology* **27**(14): 2374–2381.

3 Maat-Kievit JA, Oepkes D, Hartwig NG *et al.* (1993) A large retinoblastoma detected in a fetus at 21 weeks of gestation. *Prenatal Diagnosis* **13**(5):377–384.

4 Reulen RC, Zeegers MP, Wallace WHB *et al.* (2009) Pregnancy Outcomes among Adult Survivors of Childhood Cancer in the British Childhood Cancer Survivor Study. *Cancer Epidemiology Biomarkers Prevention* **18**(8):2239–2247.

5 Signorello LB, Cohen SS, Bosetti C *et al.* (2006) Female survivors of childhood cancer: preterm birth and low birth weight among their children. *Journal of the National Cancer Institute* **98**(20):1453–1461.

6 Winther JF, Boice JD, Frederiksen K *et al.* (2009) Radiotherapy for childhood cancer and risk for congenital malformations in offspring: a population-based cohort study. *Clinical Genetics* **75**(1):50–56.

Tuberous sclerosis

A 23-year-old woman is referred for genetic counseling because two maternal aunts reportedly have Down syndrome. Both aunts are deceased and were institutionalized in their teens in the early 1960s.

A family history of Down syndrome is a frequent reason for referral for genetic counseling. However, the term "Down syndrome" is often used by families as a generic description for mental retardation regardless of the underlying cause. The presence of two second-degree relatives with Down syndrome raises concern that this woman may carry an inherited chromosomal translocation. Even in the absence of chromosomal information on the aunts, she needs a peripheral blood karyotype to determine whether she has an increased risk for having a child with Down syndrome above that predicted by her age. However, if the aunts did not have Down syndrome but rather some other genetic disorder, a normal karyotype for the woman would not have relevance as to whether she is at increased risk for having affected children.

Medical records of the aunts are probably no longer available, and if they were born prior to the mid 1960s, it is doubtful whether chromosomal analysis would have been performed. Descriptions of the aunts and family photographs may be of help in providing more information about their diagnosis.

Relatives provide photographs of her aunts shortly before their institutionalization. Neither appear to have the characteristic facies of Down syndrome; both have disfiguring acne-like lesions on their faces. Upon further questioning of other family members, it was revealed that one of the aunts had a seizure disorder and died of kidney disease in her 30s. The other aunt died of a brain tumor in her 40s.

Based on this information, the diagnosis of Down syndrome in the maternal aunts is extremely unlikely. The aunts likely have a genetic syndrome but establishing their diagnosis with such limited information can be problematic. If they have a single gene disorder, autosomal recessive and autosomal dominant inheritance would be the most likely possibilities. If the former, the risk of occurrence of their disorder in the women's children would be small, presuming that she is unrelated to her husband. If the latter, the risk could be considerable because autosomal dominant disorders very often have a wide range of clinical expression even among members of the same family. Some affected relatives have such subtle findings that they go undiagnosed. The recognized abnormalities of the aunts (i.e., skin lesions, seizures, mental retardation, brain tumor) could be entered into a genetics database and might help narrow the differential diagnosis. In light of the aunts' histories, a complete pedigree analysis and genetics evaluation of the woman and her mother are recommended.

The woman and her mother are evaluated by a medical geneticist and the pedigree is expanded. The mother's first child, an older brother of the woman, was born in another country and died in the first few weeks of life of a rare heart tumor. Both the woman and her mother have normal intelligence and deny any major medical problems. Physical examination of the mother reveals a few hypopigmented macules on her skin. The daughter's examination also shows hypopigmented macules as well as facial

angiofibromas which the woman reports have been present for several years and were previously diagnosed by the woman's primary care doctor as acneiform lesions for which treatment with retinoic acid was prescribed.

The presence of three or more hypopigmented macules and facial angiofibromas does meet clinical criteria for a definitive diagnosis of tuberous sclerosis complex. The aunts' clinical descriptions and photographs, and the brother who probably had a cardiac tumor, also support this diagnosis.

Tuberous sclerosis is an autosomal dominant multisystem disorder which displays a high degree of clinical variability within and among families. The disorder is characterized by a number of different dermatologic findings, brain abnormalities including cortical tubers, subependymal nodules, seizures and mental retardation, renal angiomyolipomas and cysts, and cardiac rhabdomyomas and arrhythmias. Central nervous system abnormalities are the leading cause of premature death in tuberous sclerosis. Renal, heart and lung abnormalities may also be associated with significant morbidity and shortened lifespan.

Mental retardation is common in tuberous sclerosis and is present in about half of affected individuals. Central nervous system tumors including cortical tubers and subependymal glial nodules occur in up to 90% of individuals who carry a disease-causing mutation, and 80% have a seizure disorder of variable severity. Almost half of individuals with a disease-causing mutation meet the diagnostic criteria for autistic spectrum disorder.

Based on a clinical diagnosis of tuberous sclerosis, the risk of recurrence in each of the woman's children is 50%. A recurring theme in genetic counseling of dominant inheritance with variable expression is that predictions about the severity of disease in a child are not possible to make. Given the diagnosis of tuberous sclerosis complex, imaging of the woman's chest, kidneys, and brain are recommended. Early detection of astrocytomas, renal angiomyolipomas, and lymphangioleiomyomatosis may lead to treatment that ameliorates some of the serious complications of tuberous sclerosis.

The woman is considering pregnancy and wants prenatal diagnosis of tuberous sclerosis.

Tuberous sclerosis can arise from a mutation in either of two genes, *TSC1* or *TSC2*. About 80% of affected individuals who have a family history of the disorder will have an identifiable mutation in one of these genes. Although further locus heterogeneity is not suspected for tuberous sclerosis, not all *TSC1* and *TSC2* gene mutations can be found in affected individuals due to the size and complexity of these genes and current limitations of the technology. Preimplantation and prenatal genetic diagnosis would both be available to the woman if a disease-causing mutation were found in one of her *TSC1* or *TSC2* genes.

Further reading

1 Crino PB, Nathanson KL, Henske EP (2006) The tuberous sclerosis complex. *New England Journal of Medicine* **355**:1345–1356.

2 Northrup H, Kit Sing Au (updated 5/7/2009) Tuberous Sclerosis Complex. In: *GeneReviews* at GeneTests: Medical Genetics Information Resource (database online). Copyright, University of Washington, Seattle. 1997–2009. Available at http://www.genetests.org. Accessed September 2009

3 Schwartz RA, Fernández G, Kotulska K *et al.* (2007) Tuberous sclerosis complex: advances in diagnosis, genetics, and management. *Journal of the American Academy of Dermatology* **57**(2):189–202.

4 Verhoef S, Bakker L, Tempelaars AM *et al.* (1999) High rate of mosaicism in tuberous sclerosis complex. *American Journal of Human Genetics* **64**:1632–1637.

Autosomal recessive disorders

Features of autosomal recessive inheritance

1 The disorder is expressed when the abnormal gene is present on both homologous autosomal chromosomes (homozygosity or compound heterozygosity for an abnormal allele).
2 The risk of recurrence is 25% when both parents are heterozygous carriers.
3 Males and females are equally likely to be affected.
4 Heterozygotes are typically unaffected.
5 Affected individuals are typically restricted to individuals in the same sibship. More than one generation may be affected in consanguineous families or when the condition has a high prevalence in the general population. The rarer the disorder, the more likely the parents are to be consanguineous.
6 Disease expression (phenotype) tends to be similar ("breeds true") among affected siblings.
7 Unaffected siblings of an affected individual have a 2/3 chance of being heterozygous for the disorder.

Congenital adrenal hyperplasia

Case 1 A woman is referred at 6 weeks' gestation because she has a 3-year-old son who is reported to have congenital adrenal hyperplasia. He was diagnosed at 2 weeks of age after hospitalization for dehydration and vomiting and requires treatment with mineralocorticoids and glucocorticoids. She wants to know the risk of recurrence of her son's condition and whether prenatal diagnosis can prevent some of the complications of the disorder.

Congenital adrenal hyperplasia (CAH) refers to a group of autosomal recessive disorders associated with varying degrees of adrenal insufficiency and, in some cases, abnormalities of sexual differentiation. These disorders result from defects in genes controlling the synthesis of cortisol from cholesterol by the adrenal cortex. The most common form is 21-hydroxylase deficiency (21-OHD) which accounts for about 95% of cases. Less common forms include lipoid congenital adrenal hyperplasia, 17α-hydroxylase deficiency, 3β-hydroxysteroid dehydrogenase deficiency, and 11β-hydroxylase deficiency.

More specific information is needed about the son's diagnosis.

Review of the son's medical record indicates that he has 21-hydroxylase deficiency (21-OHD), diagnosed shortly after birth after a salt-wasting crisis. He has had no further medical problems since appropriate hormonal replacement was initiated and he is developing normally.

The classic form of 21-OHD is associated with severe adrenal insufficiency and very often with salt-losing crises in the first days or weeks of life. In addition, in utero exposure to excessive fetal androgens can lead to varying degrees of genital ambiguity in females due to virilization of the female genitalia. In severe cases, complete labioscrotal fusion and phallic urethra formation occurs. Effects of excessive androgen exposure on subsequent sexual orientation in affected females are also suspected. The classic form of the disorder can also present during the toddler years with early virilization without salt-wasting. In females, the non-classic or mild form of the disorder may be asymptomatic or present with hirsutism and menstrual irregularity during adolescence or with early puberty or sexual precocity in school-age children.

The patient is concerned about the high probability that an affected female fetus will be virilized.

Because 21-OHD is an autosomal recessive disorder, risk of an affected female fetus is 1 in 8 ($^1/_2$ chance that the fetus is female × $^1/_4$ chance that the fetus is affected).

Prenatal diagnosis of 21-OHD can be accomplished by analysis of DNA obtained from chorionic villi or amniocytes if the disease-causing mutations in the causative gene (*CYP21A2*) have been identified. More than 90% of *CYP21A2* gene mutations are identifiable with current laboratory methods. DNA was collected from the patient, her husband and the affected son for mutation testing.

Glucocorticoid (dexamethasone) treatment of the mother can prevent or lessen the severity of virilization of the external genitalia of affected female fetuses, thereby reducing the need for postnatal genital reconstructive surgery. Virilization of the affected female begins as early as 5 menstrual weeks' gestation. Thus, treatment of the mother should be considered as soon as the pregnancy is recognized. Short-term adverse effects of treatment on maternal health include increased appetite with weight gain, signs of Cushing syndrome, and psychological symptoms. No serious persistent adverse effects on maternal or fetal health have been reported in association with maternal glucocorticoid therapy; however, long-term follow-up studies have not been carried out. Prenatal treatment of the mother with dexamethasone does not eliminate the need for postnatal treatment of an affected child.

Treatment of the mother should be continued until the fetal sex and disease status have been established by chorionic villus sampling. If chorionic villus sampling shows that the fetus is an affected female, treatment of the mother should continue for the duration of the pregnancy. Because the safety of maternal treatment with dexamethasone has not been established and questions have been raised about adverse effects on the mother and/or fetus, treatment should be managed by endocrinologists with expertise in CAH and maternal fetal medicine specialists. Current practice is to discontinue steroid treatment except in the case of an affected female fetus.

The mother is referred to an endocrinologist and placed on dexamethasone therapy pending the results of chorionic villus sampling.

The results of molecular analysis of DNA obtained from peripheral blood leucocytes of the affected son, his mother, and father become available at 9 weeks' gestation. The affected son is a compound heterozygote for two "severe" mutations causing his classic disease. His father is heterozygous for one of those mutations. His mother carries two mutations, a "severe" mutation which she transmitted to her son, and another "mild" mutation known to be associated with the non-classic disease.

The results of DNA analysis are consistent with the son's clinical diagnosis of severe disease. An unexpected finding is that the mother also has CAH. Her physical examination is remarkable only for facial hirsutism. She has had no medical or fertility problems.

Because disease-causing mutations have been identified in this family, definitive prenatal diagnosis of CAH is possible by analysis of DNA obtained from uncultured chorionic villi in this and future pregnancies. Preimplantation genetic diagnosis would also be possible for a future pregnancy. The mother should be referred to an endocrinologist for evaluation. Although she may be asymptomatic throughout her entire life, there may be situations in which she may require treatment with glucocorticoids.

The fetus has a 25% risk of inheriting each of the parents' "severe" mutations. The fetus also has an additional 25% risk of inheriting the father's "severe" mutation and the mother's "mild" mutation. If the fetus inherits two "severe" mutations, classic salt-wasting disease as seen in the son would be predicted. However, predictions about the severity of disease will be more

difficult to make if the fetus inherits the father's "severe" mutation and the mother's "mild" mutation.

In general, compound heterozygotes for a "severe" and a "mild" *CYP21A2* mutation usually have clinical expression which is associated with the less severe of the two gene mutations. In the above case, this would predict mild disease as the mother appears to be asymptomatic other than facial hirsutism. However, caution about this conclusion is warranted because the phenotype does not always correlate precisely with the genotype and because other as yet unrecognized genes are also thought to influence clinical manifestations of the disorder.

If chorionic villus sampling reveals that the fetus is female and has inherited two "severe" alleles, dexamethasone treatment of the mother should be continued for the duration of the pregnancy. If the fetus is a compound heterozygote for a "severe" and a "mild" mutation, continued treatment with dexamethasone should be given serious consideration because the possibility of severe disease cannot be excluded. Published experience with the specific mutations in other individuals with the same genotype might help with clinical management in this circumstance.

The accuracy of the results of DNA analysis of chorionic villi is over 99%. Nonetheless, because CAH is a life-threatening disorder in the newborn period, the results of DNA analysis predicting an unaffected fetus should be confirmed immediately after birth by the measurement of serum 17-hydroxyprogesterone. In a baby who is known to be at high risk for CAH based on family history, relying on newborn screening for assessment of disease status is not sufficient.

Case 2 A 29-year-old woman and her husband are seen by a fertility specialist after 3 years of infertility. The woman successfully conceives a pregnancy by in vitro fertilization. As part of the infertility evaluation, the woman is found to have an elevated level of 17-hydroxyprogesterone in her serum and is diagnosed with a mild form of congenital adrenal hyperplasia due to 21-hydroxylase deficiency. She reports menstrual irregularity and acne as a teenager. She has no medical problems. She is referred at 5 weeks' gestation for consultation regarding the risk of congenital adrenal hyperplasia in the current pregnancy.

The woman may have two "mild" *CYP21A2* gene mutations or she may have a "mild" and a "severe" mutation. The chance that her husband is a carrier of a *CYP21A2* gene mutation needs to be established in order to determine the risk of an affected fetus.

The incidence of the classic form of congenital adrenal hyperplasia varies according to ethnicity. Among northern Europeans including Eastern European (Ashkenazi) Jews, the incidence is about 1 in 14 000 while among African Americans the incidence is 1 in 42 000. The nonclassic form of CAH is one of the most common autosomal recessive disorders with an incidence ranging from 1 in 100 to 1 in 1000 in most populations. An even higher incidence is seen in Hispanics, Ashkenazi Jews, and Mediterraneans. Among Ashkenazi Jews the incidence of the mild form is 1 in 27. Many females and most males with the mild form of CAH go undiagnosed.

| *The husband is of Ashkenazi Jewish descent.*

The chance that the husband carries a "severe" *CYP21A2* gene mutation is 1 in 60 [calculated using the Hardy–Weinberg equilibrium ($p^2 + 2pq + q^2 = 1$) where $q^2 = 1$ in 14 000], and where $p + q = 1$ (See page 39 also). The chance that the husband carries at least one "mild" *CYP21A2* gene mutation is at least 1 in 3.2 [calculated using the Hardy–Weinberg equilibrium where $q^2 = 1$ in 27]. It is this high because of the high carrier frequency of "mild" mutations among Ashkenazi Jews.

In order to calculate the possibility of classic CAH in the fetus, several possible genotypes of both parents must be considered as there are a number of scenarios that could be present. The mother could have two "mild" *CYP21A2* gene mutations, or she could have a "mild" and a "severe" mutation. The father could be a carrier of at least one mild mutation (his chance is 1 in 3.2) or he could be a carrier of a "severe" mutation (his chance is 1 in 60). Although less likely, the father could also have two "mild" mutations or have both a "mild" and a "severe" mutation.

If the mother has two "mild" mutations, the fetus would be an obligate carrier for at least one "mild" mutation. In this case, the risk of the fetus having two "mild" mutations would be 1 in 6.4 [1 (the mother's chance of transmitting a "mild" mutation) × 1 in 3.2 (the father's chance of carrying a "mild" mutation) × ¹/₂ (the chance that the father transmits his "mild" mutation to the fetus]. The risk of the fetus inheriting a "mild" mutation from the mother and inheriting a "severe" mutation from the father would be 1 in 120 [1 (the mother's chance of transmitting a "mild" mutation) × 1 in 60 (the father's chance of carrying a "severe" mutation) × ¹/₂ (the chance that the father transmits his "severe" mutation to the fetus)]. In this situation, the fetus could have classic disease

although mild CAH would be the more likely outcome. Complete phenotypic predictions before birth are not possible.

If the woman has a "mild" and a "severe" mutation, then there would be a chance of the fetus being homozygous for two "severe" mutations and having the classic form of CAH. This risk would be 1 in 240 [¹/₂ (the mother's chance of transmitting her "severe" mutation) × 1 in 60 (the father's chance of carrying a "severe" mutation) × ¹/₂ (the chance that the father transmits his "severe" mutation to the fetus)].

More than 90% of *CYP21A2* gene mutations can be detected by current laboratory methods. Analysis of the parents' DNA can be accomplished quickly to determine whether there is a risk of classic disease and whether prenatal diagnosis by chorionic villus sampling is indicated. In the meantime, the mother can be treated with dexamethasone to prevent virilization of a female fetus with classic disease.

Prompt evaluation of the newborn by measurement of 17-hydroxyprogesterone should be accomplished in all situations where a parent is known to be affected, even with mild disease.

Further reading

1 Krone N, Arlt W (2009) Genetics of congenital adrenal hyperplasia. *Best Practice and Research Clinical Endocrinology and Metabolism* **23**(2):181–192.
2 New M, Nimkarn S (Updated 9/7/2007). 21-Hydroxylase-Deficient Congenital Adrenal Hyperplasia. In: *GeneReviews* at GeneTests: Medical Genetics Information Resource (database online). Copyright, University of Washington, Seattle. 1997–2009. Available at http://www.genetests.org. Accessed September 2009.
3 Nimkarn S, New MI (2009) Prenatal diagnosis and treatment of congenital adrenal hyperplasia due to 21-hydroxylase deficiency. *Molecular and Cellular Endocrinology* **300**(1–2):192–196.
4 Speiser PW (2009) Non-classic adrenal hyperplasia. *Reviews in Endocrine and Metabolic Disorders* **10**(1): 77–82.

Cystic fibrosis

Case 1 *A couple of northern European ancestry comes for genetic counseling to discuss the results of cystic fibrosis gene testing and the risk of the disorder in their current pregnancy. The wife, who is a long-distance runner, is heterozygous for the R117H mutation in the CFTR gene.*

Her husband, who is also an athlete, is heterozygous for the common ΔF508 mutation. Testing of the couple's polymorphisms in the intron 8 polythymidine tract of the CFTR gene shows that the mother is homozygous for the 7T allele and the father is heterozygous for the 7T and 9T alleles. The couple has a 4-year-old daughter who is < 5th centile for height and weight, has severe chronic sinusitis, evidence of opacification of the sinus membranes on CT scan, tear duct stenosis bilaterally, and normal motor and cognitive development. She is heterozygous for ΔF508. The couple's son has normal cognitive and motor development and does not carry either of the parents' cystic fibrosis gene mutations. Both children have had negative sweat tests. The family history also includes the husband's brother's son who also reportedly carries the ΔF508 mutation and had pancreatitis at age 4 years.

The couple has a 25% risk in each pregnancy of a fetus who is a compound heterozygote for ΔF508/R117H. The ΔF508 mutation, which accounts for about 70% of CFTR gene mutations among Caucasians, is a "severe" CFTR mutation and in the homozygous form is usually associated with a classic cystic fibrosis presentation. The R117H mutation (in the absence of a 5T variant in *cis*) is a "mild" mutation and in combination with ΔF508 on the other homologous chromosome is associated with a wide range of phenotypes including entirely asymptomatic, milder late-onset presentation, or severe disease. Making predictions for this couple is complicated by the information we have about their daughter which is suggestive of a cystic fibrosis-like disorder despite her having inherited only her father's cystic fibrosis mutation. This raises the possibility that the mother, despite her lack of symptoms, is a compound heterozygote for two cystic fibrosis mutations, only one of which was detected by routine mutation screening. In contrast to mutation screening which only detects common CFTR gene mutations, gene sequencing will find about 99% of CFTR gene mutations.

Cystic fibrosis gene sequencing is indicated for the daughter. In addition to ΔF508, she is found to have a rare cystic fibrosis mutation, L346P, which in other families has been reported in association with mild disease. Further testing of the family showed that the mother also carries this rare mutation and confirms that the daughter is a compound heterozygote for ΔF508/L346P.

It is now possible to explain the discrepancies in the phenotypes of the daughter and father. The father carries only one cystic fibrosis mutation and does not have manifestations of the disorder. In contrast, the daughter has inherited a "severe" mutation from her father and a "mild" mutation from her mother resulting in an intermediate phenotype in which some symptoms of cystic fibrosis are present at an early age. The mother is very unusual in that she carries two "mild" mutations in the CFTR gene and has no apparent symptoms of the disease. As she is a long-distance runner, we can assume she has normal pulmonary function. Whether she is at increased risk for developing later-onset atypical manifestations of cystic fibrosis including bronchiectasis and pancreatitis is not known.

With respect to future children, the couple has a 50% chance of having a child who is a compound heterozygote for two cystic fibrosis mutations (ΔF508/R117H or ΔF508/L346P). While published reports indicate that individuals with the ΔF508/L346P genotype usually have a milder phenotype, definitive predictions for the couple's children cannot be made.

Case 2   A couple of Ashkenazi Jewish ancestry wants information about the risk of cystic fibrosis in a future pregnancy. The wife had a sister who died at age 18 years of complications of cystic fibrosis. She had severe pulmonary disease and pancreatic insufficiency. The husband has no family history of the disorder. Cystic fibrosis gene mutation screening shows that the husband is heterozygous for the W1282X mutation in the CFTR gene which is the most common CFTR gene mutation seen in Ashkenazi Jews and is usually associated with severe disease. The wife does not carry one of the 25 common cystic fibrosis mutations included in the screening panel. These 25 mutations account for 97% of mutations found in Ashkenazi Jews.

Because the wife had a sister who had cystic fibrosis, the wife's a priori risk of being a cystic fibrosis mutation carrier is 2/3. The wife's sister had classic cystic fibrosis making it likely that she had two "severe" mutations which would be included in the common mutation screening panel, but there remains a small chance that the sister had at least one rare mutation which is not detected by routine screening.

Because the wife does not carry a common cystic fibrosis mutation, her calculated residual risk of being a carrier has been reduced to 1 in 18. This Bayesian analysis takes into consideration the woman's a priori risk of 2/3 and the 97% detection rate in Ashkenazi Jewish individuals for the common mutations which were included in the mutation screening panel. The residual risk of a child affected by cystic fibrosis is 1 in 72 [1 (the chance that the husband is a carrier) $\times$ $^1/_2$ (the chance of transmission of this allele) $\times$ 1 in 18 (the chance that the wife is a carrier) $\times$ $^1/_2$ (the chance that she transmits the allele)].

The couple still faces a significant risk of having a child with cystic fibrosis. Although the wife does not carry a common identifiable CFTR gene mutation, there is a small chance that her sister had one (or two) less common cystic fibrosis mutations which were not included in the screening panel and for which the wife was not tested.

In the absence of a living affected family member, there are two approaches that could be used in this situation to provide more information about the wife. She could have gene sequencing which will detect about 99% of cystic fibrosis mutations. A negative result (i.e., no cystic fibrosis mutation detected) would further reduce her carrier risk to about 1 in 50 and the risk of an affected child to about 1 in 200. In the wife's situation, a better alternative to gene sequencing is available. Her parents, who are obligate carriers of a *CFTR* gene mutation, are living. Screening them for the presence of common cystic fibrosis mutations has a good chance of providing more information given that their affected daughter had classic disease.

The wife's parents have cystic fibrosis mutation screening. Her mother is a ΔF508 heterozygote and her father is a W1282X heterozygote.

The results of the wife's parents' cystic fibrosis mutation screening tests allow definitive information to be given to the wife. She did not inherit either of her parents' cystic fibrosis mutations and is almost certainly not a carrier of a *CFTR* gene mutation. The risk of cystic fibrosis in her children is negligible.

Case 3 *A couple is referred for counseling about in vitro fertilization and intracytoplasmic sperm injection. The couple had a 3-year history of infertility. A fertility evaluation revealed the husband has azoospermia due to congenital bilateral absence of the vas deferens. He is otherwise in good health. Subsequent analysis revealed he is heterozygous for ΔF508. His intron 8 polythymidine status is 5T/9T. The wife is heterozygous for the G542X mutation in the CFTR gene which is a classic "severe" mutation and is 7T/7T in her intron 8 polythymidine tract.*

Polymorphisms in the intron 8 polythymidine tract of the *CFTR* gene are known to influence disease expression.

The tract may have 5, 7, or 9 thymidines. The 5T variant may be associated with significantly decreased transcription of the functional cystic fibrosis gene. It has clinical importance when it is present in *trans* with a *CFTR* gene mutation or another 5T variant (i.e., there is 5T variant on one chromosome 7 and there is a *CFTR* gene mutation or another 5T tract on the homologous chromosome). Population studies show that the ΔF508 mutation occurs almost exclusively on chromosomes with the 9T variant (i.e., the 9T variant is in *cis* with ΔF508).

Congenital bilateral absence of the vas deferens (CBAVD) in an otherwise healthy infertile man has a significant chance of being explained by one or more mutations in the *CFTR* gene. About two-thirds of such men will be compound heterozygotes for two cystic fibrosis mutations or have at least one cystic fibrosis mutation, and almost half will also have the intron 8 5T variant. In contrast, only about 5% of the general population carries a 5T allele. For this reason, cystic fibrosis mutation testing is indicated for all men with CBAVD because they have a significant chance of transmitting a cystic fibrosis mutation to their offspring, which in combination with a mutant maternal allele could result in a more severe phenotype.

In this couple's pregnancy, the fetus has a 25% chance of being a compound heterozygote for ΔF508/G542X which is associated with severe pulmonary disease and pancreatic insufficiency.

The fetus also has a 25% chance of inheriting G542X from the mother and the intron 8 5T variant from the father. This combination is associated with varying clinical phenotypes ranging from no significant symptomatology to absent vas deferens, chronic or recurrent upper airway disease (bronchi, sinuses, middle ear), asthma, chronic or recurrent pancreatitis, or classic childhood cystic fibrosis. The spectrum of clinical phenotypes is presumably due to differing effects on CFTR transcription from the cystic fibrosis gene on the chromosome that has the 5T variant and other epigenetic or post-translational processes. It is not possible to give predictions about the phenotype aside from frequency observations that suggest that milder phenotypes are more common than severe ones.

Case 4 *Cystic fibrosis carrier testing reveals that a woman carries a R117H cystic fibrosis mutation. Her poly T status in intron 8 of the CFTR gene is 5T/7T. Her husband does not carry one of the 97 CFTR gene mutations tested for by a commercial screening panel. His poly T status in intron 8* *is 7T/7T. The husband's ancestry is half Korean and half northern European. The wife has chorionic villus sampling because she is 40 years old and elects to establish the fetal CFTR gene status. Analysis of DNA obtained from un-cultured chorionic villi indicates that the fetus inherited the patient's R117H CFTR mutation. The fetal poly T variant status in intron 8 is 5T/7T. The fetus is heterozygous for both R117H and the 5T variant.*

The father had to transmit the 7T allele, thus the results of prenatal diagnosis have also established that the wife's R117H mutation and her 5T variant in intron 8 are in *cis*, i.e., on the same chromosome. The presence of the R117H mutation on the same chromosome as the 5T variant results in a severe mutation. If the fetus inherited another cystic fibrosis mutation on the other copy of chromosome number 7 inherited from the husband, this could be associated with severe disease.

The husband is of half-Asian ancestry where the sensitivity of mutation screening for common mutations is decreased compared to individuals of European ancestry. There is still incomplete knowledge of the spectrum of cystic fibrosis mutations and carrier frequencies seen in various Asian populations. The negative results of his cystic fibrosis carrier testing are estimated to reduce the husband's risk of being a carrier to less than 1 in 100. The residual risk of the cystic fibrosis spectrum of disorders in the current pregnancy is about 1 in 200 although the risk is probably smaller as the calculation conservatively assumes that *CFTR* mutation screening has a very low mutation detection rate among persons with Asian ancestry.

The option of further cystic fibrosis mutation analysis by DNA sequencing of the husband is a consideration if the family wants more information, because DNA sequencing will find almost all clinically important cystic fibrosis mutations regardless of ancestral background. However, predictions about the severity of symptoms in a child if the husband carries a rare cystic fibrosis mutation may be difficult. Although a mild rather than severe disorder would be more likely, the symptoms of cystic fibrosis that could be present in a child who inherited his mother's R117H mutation and a rare mutation from his father would include chronic progressive lung disease, pancreatic insufficiency, less severe respiratory and sinus disease, and male infertility. Predictions about the severity of symptoms for any given individual would not be possible to make. However, in this couple's pregnancy with the information available from prenatal diagnosis,

the most likely outcome will be a baby who does not have the cystic fibrosis spectrum of disease.

Further reading

1 Chillón M, Casals T, Mercier B *et al.* (1995) Mutations in the cystic fibrosis gene in patients with congenital absence of the vas deferens. *New England Journal of Medicine* **332**(22):1475–1480.

2 Cohn JA, Friedman KJ, Noone PG *et al.* (1998) Relation between mutations of the cystic fibrosis gene and idiopathic pancreatitis. *New England Journal of Medicine* **339**(10):653–658.

3 Gallati S (2003) Genetics of cystic fibrosis. *Seminars in Respiratory and Critical Care Medicine* **24**(6):629–638.

4 Kanavakis E, Tzetis M, Antoniadi T *et al.* (1998) Cystic fibrosis mutation screening in CBAVD patients and men with obstructive azoospermia or severe oligozoospermia. *Molecular Human Reproduction* **4**(4):333–337.

5 Kerem E (2006) Atypical CF and CF related diseases. *Paediatric Respiratory Reviews* 7 **Suppl 1**:S144–146.

6 Lebo RV, Omlor GJ (2007) Targeted extended cystic fibrosis mutation testing on known and at-risk patients and relatives. *Genetic Testing* **11**(4):427–444.

7 Moskowitz SM, Chmiel JF, Sternen DL *et al.* (2008) Clinical practice and genetic counseling for cystic fibrosis and CFTR-related disorders. *Genetics in Medicine* **10**(12):851–868.

8 Rowntree RK, Harris A (2003) The phenotypic consequences of CFTR mutations. *Annals of Human Genetics* **67**(Pt 5):471–485.

Spinal muscular atrophy

Case 1 A couple of northern European ancestry is concerned about the risk of spinal muscular atrophy in their current pregnancy because a neighbor's child was recently diagnosed with the severe infantile form.

Spinal muscular atrophy (SMA) is a common autosomal recessive condition among Caucasians with an incidence of about 1 in 5000. As seen in cystic fibrosis, the disease incidence varies among different ethnic groups as shown in Table 2.1. SMA is associated with progressive muscle weakness due to degeneration of the anterior horn cells in the spinal cord and brainstem nuclei. There is a wide range of disease severity associated with the same underlying molecular defects which has been categorized into separate types of SMA. It is

Table 2.1 Carrier frequency and risk reductions for individuals who have no family history of SMA

Ethnicity	A priori carrier risk	Disease incidence	Carrier detection rate	Reduced carrier risk when two copies of *SMN1* are present
Caucasian	1 : 35	1 : 4900	94.9%	1 : 632
Ashkenazi Jewish	1 : 41	1 : 6700	90.2%	1 : 350
Asian	1 : 53	1 : 11 200	92.6%	1 : 628
Hispanic	1 : 117	1 : 55 000	90.6%	1 : 1061
African American	1 : 66	1 : 17 500	71.1%	1 : 121

Data from Hendrickson BC, Donohoe C, Akmaev VR *et al.* (2009) *Journal of Medical Genetics* **46**:641–644.

important to recognize that the spectrum of symptoms represents a disease continuum rather than discrete clinical entities.

The most common form, comprising about 70% of cases, is SMA type 1 (also known as Werdnig–Hoffman disease) in which symptoms become apparent before 6 months with progressive swallowing and sucking difficulties. Death from respiratory failure usually occurs within two years in the absence of aggressive respiratory support. SMA type 2 is associated with onset of symptoms after 6 months of age. Affected individuals are not ambulatory but are able to sit without support if placed in a sitting position. Symptoms of SMA type 3 usually begin after 10 months. Severe muscle weakness is present but ambulation for short distances is usually possible. Type 0 has a prenatal onset where clinical features may include polyhydramnios, fetal akinesia, and arthrogryposis.

Using the Hardy–Weinberg equilibrium, the carrier frequency for an autosomal recessive disorder can be derived from the disease incidence if it is known. Among northern Europeans, the disease incidence is 1 in 4900.

$$p = \text{frequency of normal allele;}$$
$$q = \text{frequency of mutant allele}$$
$$q^2 = \text{disease incidence}$$
$$p + q = 1$$
$$p^2 + 2pq + q^2 = 1$$
$$2pq = \text{carrier frequency}$$
$$q^2 = 1/4900$$
$$q = 1 \text{ in } 70; \; p \text{ is approximately } 1$$

$2pq = 1$ in 35 (this is the chance that someone in the general population without a family history of the disorder will be a carrier for SMA)

All forms of SMA are due to mutations in the *SMN1* (survival motor neuron 1) gene located on chromosome 5q. Ninety-five to 98% of affected individuals are homozygous for a deletion of exons 7 and 8 of *SMN1*. Most of the remaining affected individuals are compound heterozygotes for a deletion of exons 7 and 8 and a point mutation in the *SMN1* gene.

Currently available carrier testing for SMA by molecular analysis looks only for the common deletion of exons 7 and 8 of the *SMN1* gene and thus will not find all carriers. Among Caucasians, about 6% of carriers will not be identified because they have a *SMN1* gene point mutation which is not detected by deletion testing, or they have a *SMN1* deletion on one chromosome which is masked by a duplication (or triplication) of exons 7 and 8 of the *SMN1* gene on the homologous chromosome as shown in Figure 2.1. Among other ancestral backgrounds, the common exon 7 and 8 deletion is less common and testing for the common deletion has a lower sensitivity in finding carriers of SMA (ranging from 71% among African Americans to almost 93% among Asians) as shown in Table 2.1.

If one member of a Caucasian couple does not carry the common *SMN1* gene deletion, that person's residual risk of being a SMA gene carrier is about 1 in 630. The residual risk of spinal muscular atrophy in the pregnancy would be about 1 in 88 000 [1/630 (the risk of being a *SMN1* mutation carrier if the person does not carry the common *SMN1* gene deletion) × $^1/_2$ (the chance of transmission of this allele) × 1/35 (the population risk for being an *SMN1* gene mutation) × $^1/_2$ (the chance of transmission of this allele)].

The variable phenotype observed in SMA can be in part accounted for by the number of copies of a nearby gene, *SMN2*, which is nearly identical to *SMN1* but produces about 10% of the protein that the *SMN1* gene produces. In the setting of a fetus who has zero copies of *SMN1* (i.e., affected by SMA), the *SMN2* copy number present in the fetus may help with predictions about disease severity. However, phenotypic predictions using *SMN2* copy number should be made cautiously because there is a

Not detectable by copy number screening

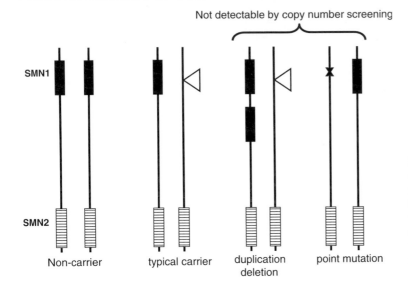

Figure 2.1 Spinal muscular atrophy gene mutations. Each pair of homologous chromosomes is shown by a pair of lines. The filled in box indicates the wild type copy of the SMN1 gene, the triangle indicates the deletion of exons 7 and 8 of the SMN1 gene, the X represents a point mutation in the SMN1 gene. The hatched box indicates the SMN2 gene.

continuum of disease expression at any *SMN2* copy number. High *SMN2* copy numbers may somewhat compensate for the absence of *SMN1* and in general, but not always, correlate with milder disease. For example, five or more copies of *SMN2* has been reported to completely compensate for absence of *SMN1* in some individuals (i.e., a normal phenotype) but still be associated with severe disease (i.e., unable to sit unsupported) in others. At lower numbers of *SMN2* copies (i.e., one, two, or three copies of *SMN2*), a wide range of disease severity is possible with severe disease being much more likely than mild. There presumably are other modifying factors, genetic or otherwise, which also play a role in disease severity.

Case 2 A couple of northern European ancestry is seen for consultation because the wife's sister had a son who recently died in infancy of spinal muscular atrophy, as shown in Figure 2.2. They want to know the risk of spinal muscular atrophy in their current pregnancy.

Before providing this woman with information about risk of occurrence of spinal muscular atrophy in her own pregnancy, it is important to confirm that the diagnosis of her nephew is correct. Several disorders have symptoms which might be mistaken for the infantile form of spinal muscular atrophy as shown in Table 2.2. Carrier testing for SMA is readily available, but a negative analysis could result in misleading and incorrect risk assessment if the diagnosis of the nephew is not confirmed.

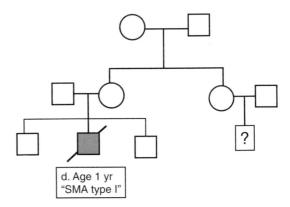

d. Age 1 yr
"SMA type I"

Figure 2.2 Pedigree of family with spinal muscular atrophy.

Since the nephew died recently, there is a good chance that his clinical diagnosis was confirmed by molecular testing of his survival motor neuron (SMN) genes. In the absence of molecular testing, as much clinical information as possible about the nephew should be reviewed.

The results of the nephew's molecular testing are obtained. He is homozygous for deletions of exons 7 and 8 in his *SMN1* genes, confirming his clinical diagnosis.

It is now possible to provide more information to the couple about their risk of having a similarly affected child.

In this couple's case, the chance that the husband is a carrier of SMA is 1 in 35 because he does not have a family history of the disorder. Calculating the wife's chance of being a carrier must take into account her family history.

Table 2.2 A partial list of disorders with a similar clinical presentation to infantile autosomal recessive SMA

Recessive SMA
  SMA + pontocerebellar hypoplasia
  Lethal congenital contracture syndrome
  Pontocerebellar hypoplasia type 1
  Spinal muscular atrophy with respiratory distress type 1 (SMARD1)
  Ullrich congenital muscular dystrophy
  Infantile acid maltase deficiency
  Nemaline myopathy
  Prader–Willi syndrome (severe hypotonia)
  Zellweger syndrome

Dominant
  Benign congenital myopathy with contractures
  Congenital myotonic dystrophy
  Autosomal dominant SMA – very rare in childhood
  Congenital benign spinal muscular atrophy

X-linked
  X-linked infant SMA + arthrogryposis
  X-linked myotubular myopathy

Mitochondrial related
  Mitochondrial complex IV deficiency

Acquired
  Congenital myasthenia gravis

Her sister, who had an affected child, is an obligate carrier of the condition. She almost certainly has a deletion of exons 7 and 8 of the *SMN* gene (discounting the small chance that her son's mutation arose from a new mutation that occurred in her ovum), and in fact, molecular testing had previously confirmed that the sister is heterozygous for this deletion.

Since (at least) one of the sister's parents must also be a carrier of the *SMN* gene mutation, the chance that our patient inherited the mutation from that parent is 50%. The risk of SMA in the couple's pregnancy is 1 in 280 [$^1/_2$ (the chance the patient is a carrier) $\times$ $^1/_2$ (the chance of transmission of this allele) $\times$ 1/35 (the chance the husband is a carrier) $\times$ $^1/_2$ (the chance of transmission of his allele)]. If both parents are carriers of *SMN1* gene mutations, definitive prenatal diagnosis by chorionic villus sampling or amniocentesis would be available, as would preimplantation genetic diagnosis.

Case 3 *A woman is concerned about the risk of spinal muscular atrophy in her current pregnancy because her brother was affected by the disorder and died of respiratory failure at age 6 months.*

The brother was noted to have hypotonia at age 2 weeks; he had facial weakness and had difficulty with sucking and swallowing. He did not reach expected motor milestones but appeared alert and smiled readily. He died before the availability of molecular testing. No other family members are reported to be affected.

Before providing this woman with information about risk of occurrence of spinal muscular atrophy in her own pregnancy, it is important to confirm that the diagnosis of her brother is correct. As discussed above, if the brother actually had some other disease, the results of DNA testing of his sister for mutations in the spinal muscular atrophy gene would not be meaningful with respect to risk of occurrence of his problems in her pregnancies.

The woman elects to have SMA carrier testing, acknowledging the limitations of molecular testing in the absence of this testing in her brother. The results of her molecular testing show that she carries two copies of the SMN1 gene.

This result needs to be interpreted cautiously because we do not have a molecular diagnosis for her brother. If her brother were affected with SMA, this analysis reduces her risk from 2/3 to 1/11. She still could be a carrier with two *SMN1* copies on one chromosome 5 and none on the other. However, the patient's parents are both alive and available for testing of their *SMN1* genes. The results of *SMN1* gene analysis show that both her parents are heterozygous for the common deletion of exons 7 and 8 in the *SMN1* gene. This information, while not proving that their son had spinal muscular atrophy, provides strong evidence to support that diagnosis. In addition, this excludes the possibility that the patient could have a deletion on one chromosome and a duplication on her other chromosome, giving the false assessment of a non-carrier. The woman can now be excluded as being a carrier for spinal muscular atrophy as she has inherited a normal *SMN1* gene from each of her parents.

Further reading

1 Hendrickson BC, Donohoe C, Akmaev VR *et al.* (2009) Differences in SMN1 allele frequencies among ethnic groups within North America. *Journal of Medical Genetics* **46**:641–644.

2 MacLeod MJ, Taylor JE, Lunt PW *et al.* (1999) Prenatal onset spinal muscular atrophy. *European Journal of Paediatric Neurology* **3**:65–72.

3 Mailman MD, Heinz JW, Papp AC *et al.* (2002) Molecular analysis of spinal muscular atrophy and modification of the phenotype of SMN2. *Genetics in Medicine* **4**(1):20–26.

4 Prior TW, Russman BS. (Updated 4/3/2006). Spinal Muscular Atrophy. In: *GeneReviews* at GeneTests: Medical Genetics Information Resource (database online). Copyright, University of Washington, Seattle. 1997–2009. Available at http://www.genetests.org. Accessed September 2009.

5 Prior TW (2007) Spinal muscular atrophy diagnostics. *Journal of Child Neurology* **22**:952–956.

6 Prior TW, Swoboda KJ, Scott HD *et al.* (2004) Homozygous SMN1 deletions in unaffected family members and modification of the phenotype by SMN2. *American Journal of Medical Genetics Part A* **130A**: 307–310.

7 Swoboda KJ, Prior TW, Scott CB *et al.* (2005) Natural history of denervation in SMA: relation to age, SMN2 copy number, and function. *Annals of Neurology* **57**:704–712.

Hemoglobinopathies

Case 1 An African American woman is referred for genetic counseling for advanced maternal age. Her husband is also African American. She elects hemoglobin variant carrier testing which shows the following:

> MCV: 68 fl. (normal range 80–100 fL)
>
> Hgb A: 92.9%
>
> Hgb A$_2$: 5.8% (normal range 1.5–3.8%)
>
> Hgb F: 1.3%

The low MCV and elevated hemoglobin A$_2$ concentration are consistent with heterozygosity for a type of beta globin gene mutation known as beta thalassemia trait. Beta thalassemia trait is seen in about 1 in 75 African Americans.

Heterozygosity for alpha and beta globin gene variants is common among African Americans as shown in Table 2.3.

This woman is at risk for having a child with beta thalassemia or hemoglobin S/beta thalassemia. The risk of beta thalassemia is 1 in 300 [1 (the chance that the woman has beta thalassemia trait) × $\frac{1}{2}$ (the chance that she transmits this mutation) × 1 in 75 (the risk that her husband is a beta thalassemia carrier) × $\frac{1}{2}$ (the chance he transmits his beta thalassemia mutation to the fetus)].

The risk of hemoglobin S/beta thalassemia is 1 in 44 [1 (the chance that the woman has beta thalassemia trait)

Table 2.3 Heterozygote frequencies for common hemoglobin variants among African Americans

Hemoglobin genotype	Incidence among African Americans
AS	1/11
AC	1/50
Beta thalassemia trait (heterozygous carrier)	1/75
Alpha thalassemia trait – deletion of 2 of 4 alpha globin genes in trans	1/30
Alpha thalassemia trait – deletion of 2 of 4 alpha globin genes in cis	rare
Alpha thalassemia trait – deletion of 1 of 4 alpha globin genes	1/3

Data from: Bunn HF, Forget BG (1986) *Hemoglobin: Molecular, Genetic and Clinical Aspects.* W.B. Saunders Company, Philadelphia.

× $\frac{1}{2}$ (chance of transmission) × 1 in 11 (the risk that her husband carries hemoglobin S) × $\frac{1}{2}$ (the chance that he transmist a beta globin gene mutation to the fetus)].

Hemoglobin variant carrier testing for the woman's husband shows that he has hemoglobin AS.

The risk of a child with hemoglobin S/beta thalassemia is 25%. Prenatal diagnosis is available by chorionic villus sampling if the woman's beta thalassemia mutation has been identified. Beta globin gene sequencing will identify most beta thalassemia mutations.

The clinical severity of hemoglobin S/beta thalassemia varies widely. Some affected individuals have only a mild or moderate anemia while others can have severe anemia, growth failure, end-organ damage, pain and disability, and other serious medical complications that are commonly seen in the usual form of sickle cell disease. It is not possible to make specific predictions for any given individual about the severity of the disease, although predictions might be influenced by the specific beta globin gene mutation carried by the woman. Some mutations, on average, are associated with a more severe anemia than others (in combination with hemoglobin S), but precise predictions would not be possible, even if information about the woman's mutation was established. Other factors influencing the degree of severity in sickle cell disease and thalassemia may include the amount of fetal hemoglobin and the alpha globin status of the individual.

Case 2 *An African American couple with the following laboratory data are referred for genetic counseling about the risks of hemoglobinopathies in the current pregnancy.*

Wife	Husband
MCV: 65.2 fL	MCV: 69.4 fL
Hct: 36%	Hct: 42%
Hgb A: 97.7%	Hgb A: 70.1%
Hgb A$_2$: 2.3%	Hgb A$_2$: 3.7%
	Hgb C: 26.2%

The laboratory data are consistent with the wife having alpha thalassemia trait with deletion of two of four alpha globin genes. Less likely possibilities include her having beta thalassemia trait because iron deficiency anemia can be associated with depressed hemoglobin A$_2$ concentration. There are also atypical cases of beta thalassemia trait which are associated with a low MCV and normal hemoglobin A$_2$ concentration.

The husband has hemoglobin C with or without alpha thalassemia trait. Hemoglobin AC can be associated with a mildly low MCV, but his microcytosis and relatively low Hgb C suggest that he may also have alpha thalassemia trait. Hemoglobin C may be co-inherited with beta thalassemia; however, these individuals have moderate to severe anemia and Hgb A levels <50%, neither of which is seen in this individual.

There is a high probability based on ethnicity (>99%) that the two alpha globin gene mutations of the wife are in the *trans* configuration (on opposite homologous chromosomes). Even if the father is also an alpha thalassemia carrier (and missing two alpha globin genes) his deletions are most probably in the *trans* configuration, thus posing a remote risk of significant fetal disease. The risk of hydrops fetalis (missing all four alpha genes) in the couple's children is less than 1 in 40 000 (1/100 × $^1/_2$ × 1/100 × $^1/_2$).

There is a small risk of hemoglobin H disease (mutations in three of the four alpha globin genes), which could occur if the husband is an alpha thalassemia gene carrier. Hemoglobin H disease is usually associated with an anemia of moderate severity.

In the unlikely event that the wife is a beta thalassemia carrier, the fetus would be at risk for having hemoglobin C/beta thalassemia. Individuals with these globin gene mutations are generally asymptomatic but may have a mild hemolytic anemia.

Because risks of clinically important alpha globin gene disorders are small in the African population, further testing to address these small risks is usually not pursued.

For a couple that wants complete information, further investigation of the couple's risk of having a child with hemoglobin H disease or hydrops fetalis would include alpha globin mutation testing of the wife and husband. If molecular analysis confirms alpha thalassemia trait in both members of the couple, family studies (testing of the couple's parents) would be needed to determine the phase of the alpha globin gene mutations (*trans* or *cis*) and whether the couple was in fact at risk for having a fetus with hydrops fetalis due to alpha thalassemia. In this highly unlikely scenario, prenatal diagnosis by chorionic villus sampling or amniocentesis could be carried out to assess the fetal alpha globin gene status.

Case 3 *A couple of Vietnamese ancestry is referred for genetic counseling about risks of hemoglobinopathies in their children. They have the following laboratory values:*

Wife	Husband
MCV: 78 fL	MCV: 64 fL
Hgb A: 60.8%	Hgb A: 93.0%
Hgb E: 38%	Hgb A$_2$: 5.7%
Hgb F: 1.2%	Hgb F: 1.3%

After alpha globin gene mutations, hemoglobin E is the most common hemoglobin variant worldwide with a prevalence of greater than 10% in some Southeast Asian populations. Hemoglobin AE and EE are clinically unimportant. However, the co-inheritance of hemoglobin E with a beta thalassemia mutation leading to absence of hemoglobin A (a beta^o thalassemia mutation) usually leads to a transfusion dependent severe anemia beginning in early childhood. Co-inheritance of hemoglobin E with a beta$^+$ thalassemia mutation in which some hemoglobin A is synthesized is usually associated with a milder anemia. This couple's laboratory data indicate that she has hemoglobin AE and he is a carrier of a beta thalassemia mutation. Their children have a 1 in 4 chance of having E/beta thalassemia disease. The husband's beta thalassemia mutation could almost certainly be determined by beta globin gene sequencing. Preimplantation or prenatal genetic diagnosis would be available for their pregnancies.

Case 4 *An African American woman is referred for genetic counseling at 20 weeks' gestation. She has hemoglobin AS. Her partner, who is also African American, is not available for hemoglobin variant testing. The woman wants prenatal diagnosis of fetal hemoglobinopathies.*

The fetus is at risk for hemoglobin SS, SC, and hemo-globin S/beta thalassemia disease with risks of 1 in 44, 1 in 200, and 1 in 300, respectively. The risks are derived from the carrier frequencies noted in Table 2.3. These risks assume that the husband is unaffected by a hemoglobin-opathy. Information about the husband's hemoglobin variant status is not necessary to provide definitive pre-natal diagnosis of hemoglobin SS and SC disease of the fetus. In contrast to most genetic disorders where a large number of different mutations can result in the same phenotype, hemoglobin S is always the result of a single nucleotide change in the beta globin gene leading to the replacement of the sixth amino acid, glutamine, by the amino acid valine in the beta globin peptide. Hemo-globin C always results from a single nucleotide change causing that same glutamine to be replaced by lysine in the beta globin peptide. Direct DNA analysis will identify these single nucleotide changes in DNA obtained from chorionic villi or amniotic fluid cells.

In contrast to hemoglobin S and C, more than 200 different mutations can lead to beta thalassemia. However, only a few mutations account for the majority of beta thalassemia carriers in each population where there is a high prevalence of the disorder and can be easily and rapidly detected by molecular testing. For example, among African Americans 75–80% of heterozygotes will have one of six beta globin gene mutations. Among individuals of Mediterranean, Chinese, Middle Eastern, Thai, and Chinese ancestry, 90–95% of beta globin mutations carriers will be detected by testing for four to six ethnic specific mutations.

Beta globin gene sequencing of DNA from a prenatal sample will identify 99% of beta globin gene mutations. Gene sequencing requires more time and at present is more expensive than targeted mutation testing.

Prenatal diagnosis of hemoglobinopathies by fetal blood sampling followed by hemoglobin electrophoresis is also technically possible but has been mostly supplanted by chorionic villus sampling or amniocentesis followed by molecular analysis, which allows for a highly accurate early prenatal diagnosis using an invasive procedure associated with lower risk to the pregnancy.

Further reading

1 Buchanan GR, DeBaun MR, Quinn CT et al. (2004) Sickle Cell Disease. *Hematology: The American Society of Hematology Education Program Book*: 35–47.
2 Bunn HF, Forget BG (1986) *Hemoglobin: Molecular, Genetic and Clinical Aspects*. W.B. Saunders Company, Philadelphia.
3 Cao A, Galanello R (Updated 10/23/2007). Beta-thalassemia. In: GeneReviews at GeneTests: Medical Genetics Information Resource (database online). Copyright, University of Washington, Seattle. 1997–2009. Available at http://www.genetests.org. Accessed September 2009.
4 Krishnamurti L, Chui DH, Dallaire M et al. (1998) Coinheritance of α-thalassemia-1 and hemoglobin E/β^0-thalassemia: practical implications for neonatal screening and genetic counseling. *Journal of Pediatrics* **132**:863–865.
5 Leung TN, Lau TK, Chung TK et al. (2005) Thalas-saemia screening in pregnancy. *Current Opinion in Obstetrics and Gynecology* **17**(2):129–134.
6 Old JM (2007) Screening and genetic diagnosis of haemoglobinopathies. *Scandinavian Journal of Clinical and Laboratory Investigation* **67**(1):71–86.
7 Sripichai O, Munkongdee T, Kumkhaek C et al. (2008) Coinheritance of the different copy numbers of alpha-globin gene modifies severity of beta-thalassemia/Hb E disease. *Annals of Hematology* **87**(5):375–379.
8 Steinberg MH, Forget, BG, Higgs, DR et al. (2001) Disorders of Hemoglobin: Genetics, Pathophysiology, and Clinical Management. Cambridge University Press, New York.
9 Winichagoon P, Fucharoen S, Chen P et al. (2000) Genetic factors affecting clinical severity in beta-thalassemia syndromes. *Journal of Pediatric Hematology/Oncology* **22**(6):573–580.

Fanconi anemia

A couple is referred at 20 weeks' gestation. They are both of Ashkenazi (eastern European) Jewish ancestry. Both members of the couple were recently found to carry a mutation in the gene associated with Fanconi anemia group C.

Fanconi anemia is an autosomal recessive disorder of chromosome instability. It is one of a group of autosomal recessive disorders that has a higher incidence among Jews of eastern European ancestry than among individuals of other ethnic backgrounds and is included in the recessive disorder screening panel which is offered to individuals of Ashkenazi Jewish background.

The clinical features of Fanconi anemia include a high chance of bone marrow failure which usually occurs in the first decade of life. Affected individuals also have a very high lifetime risk of hematopoietic malignancies and solid tumors at young ages, the latter of which may be the first sign of Fanconi anemia in some individuals. In two-thirds of affected individuals, a wide range of physical abnormalities of variable severity are present but are not usually a major source of morbidity. Treatment of bone marrow failure consists of administration of oral androgens to increase white cell, red cell, and platelet counts and administration of granulocyte colony-stimulating factor to increase white cell counts. Because Fanconi anemia is a chromosome breakage syndrome, treatment of malignancies is problematic and preparative regimens for bone marrow transplantation must be modified because affected individuals are exquisitely sensitive to the effects of ionizing radiation and chemotherapeutic agents. Allogeneic bone marrow or stem cell transplant using cells from an HLA matched donor can be curative with respect to the hematologic abnormalities of Fanconi anemia but does not reduce the significant risk of solid tumors.

Fanconi anemia is genetically heterogeneous. Mutations in 13 different genes (complementation groups) have been shown to cause Fanconi anemia. Some are associated with earlier onset of hematologic malignancies and a higher incidence of structural abnormalities. The disease state arises only in individuals who are homozygous for two mutations in the same complementation group (the same gene). Ashkenazi Jews have a higher incidence of Fanconi anemia associated with complementation group C, but not of Fanconi anemia associated with mutations in other genes. The incidence of Fanconi anemia group C in Ashkenazi Jews is 1 in 32 000 with a carrier frequency of 1 in 90.

Each of the couple's children has a 25% chance of being homozygous for the parents' Fanconi anemia mutations. Because both parents have a characterized mutation in their Fanconi anemia group C gene, definitive prenatal diagnosis is possible in the current pregnancy by analysis of DNA obtained from chorionic villi or amniocytes.

| *The couple has three other children.*

Their children should be tested to determine whether they are affected by Fanconi anemia. Some affected individuals, especially early in their lives, may go undiagnosed as they may not have hematologic or structural abnormalities. It is important that their Fanconi anemia status be established so that they can have careful surveillance for and early treatment of bone marrow failure.

Testing the children of this couple for Fanconi anemia can be accomplished by molecular analysis of DNA obtained from their peripheral blood since the disease-causing mutations in the parents are already known. Cytogenetic testing to look for increased chromosome breakage when cells are exposed to diepoxybutane, a DNA clastogenic agent, is another highly sensitive and specific method for diagnosis of Fanconi anemia and is used when the disorder is suspected and familial mutations are not known.

A son, age 4 years, was born with a duplicated thumb which was surgically corrected during infancy. He is otherwise well. A daughter, age 3, has conductive hearing loss requiring hearing aids. Another daughter age 7 has had no medical problems.

In the context of parental heterozygosity for Fanconi anemia group C gene mutations, the skeletal abnormality in the couple's son and the hearing loss in their daughter raise significant concerns that they are affected by Fanconi anemia. Upper limb malformations including absent or supernumerary thumbs are present in about 40% of affected individuals. Ear abnormalities including hearing loss are present in about 10%. The diagnosis of Fanconi anemia is sometimes missed in affected individuals with relatively minor structural abnormalities until bone marrow failure occurs.

Mutation testing is performed on the couple's children. The couple's son and their younger daughter with hearing loss are affected by Fanconi anemia. Both showed increased chromosomal breakage when their cells were exposed to diepoxybutane. The couple's older daughter is not affected. The son's CBC is abnormal; his platelets, hematocrit, and white cell count are low. The affected daughter's CBC is normal.

The only effective treatment for bone marrow failure associated with Fanconi anemia is bone marrow/stem cell transplantation from an HLA-matched sibling or other HLA-matched donor.

| *The couple's unaffected daughter has HLA typing and is not an HLA match for either of her siblings.*

The couple elects to have prenatal diagnosis of Fanconi anemia via analysis of DNA obtained from cultured amniocytes. DNA could also be obtained from chorionic villi, even at 20 weeks' gestation, if the placenta were easily accessible. Chorionic villus sampling would be the preferable procedure in this circumstance because it provides a large quantity of DNA without having to culture cells.

If the fetus is not affected by Fanconi anemia, the fetus could be a stem cell or bone marrow donor for one or both of his or her siblings if the fetus is an HLA match. Although complete matches are not a requirement for transplantation, they are associated with the highest chance of successful donor cell engraftment and the lowest risk of serious complications. The chance that two siblings have the same HLA haplotypes is 1 in 4.

In this couple's pregnancy, the chance that the fetus is unaffected by Fanconi anemia is $^3/_4$. The chance that the fetus is an identical HLA match for any given sibling is $^1/_4$.

If the fetus is unaffected by Fanconi anemia, preliminary HLA typing could be performed using DNA obtained from amniotic fluid or chorionic villus cells. If the fetus is an HLA match, cord blood banking is recommended. Stem cells from cord blood of an HLA-matched sibling could be used for stem cell transplantation of an affected sibling. If the fetus is not affected by Fanconi anemia and is not an HLA match for an affected sibling, cord blood banking should be considered if future pregnancies are contemplated and pregnancy termination of a fetus affected by Fanconi anemia is not a consideration.

For future pregnancies, preimplantation genetic diagnosis to identify embryos unaffected by Fanconi anemia group C and who are HLA matches for an affected sibling would also be possible.

Further reading

1 Green AM, Kupfer GM (2009) Fanconi anemia. *Hematology/Oncology Clinics of North America* **23**(2): 193–214.

2 Kutler DI, Auerbach AD (2004) Fanconi anemia in Ashkenazi Jews. *Familial Cancer* **3**:241–248.

3 Taniguchi T (updated 3/27/2008) Fanconi Anemia. In: *GeneReviews* at GeneTests: Medical Genetics Information Resource (database online). Copyright, University of Washington, Seattle. 1997–2009. Available at http://www.genetests.org. Accessed September 2009.

4 Verlinsky Y, Rechitsky S, Schoolcraft W *et al.* (2001) Preimplantation Diagnosis for Fanconi Anemia Combined With HLA Matching. *Journal of the American Medical Association* **285**(24):3130–3133.

Maple syrup urine disease

A woman inquires about the risk of maple syrup urine disease (MSUD) in her current pregnancy. She reports that her husband has a son and daughter from a previous marriage who are affected by the disorder and were diagnosed via newborn screening. She has no further information about these children.

MSUD is a metabolic disorder caused by decreased activity of the branched-chain alpha ketoacid dehydrogenase complex (BCKAD) which, untreated, leads to metabolic decompensation and death. Providing accurate information about the risk of occurrence of her husband's children's disorder depends on a number of factors including the accuracy of the information being provided, the mode of inheritance of the disorder, whether the family history is compatible with the diagnosis, and whether there is consanguinity between the woman and her husband or if the woman is related to her husband's previous wife.

In this scenario, the only information that is available about the affected children is that they are on a special diet, have frequent medical appointments but are generally healthy. No laboratory data is available for review. The woman appears to be a reliable historian. No other family members are known to be affected. The woman denies consanguinity with her husband and is not related to her husband's previous wife.

It is always preferable to provide information about risks of birth defects or a genetic disorder after review of medical records or discussions with the physicians caring for the affected individual. Practically, however, this is often not possible and genetic risk information is provided assuming that a particular diagnosis is correct and acknowledging the occasional serious pitfalls of this assumption.

Online Mendelian Inheritance in Man (OMIM) and GeneTests are web-based resources which provide high quality peer-reviewed information about genetic disorders. A review of OMIM shows that MSUD has autosomal recessive inheritance. The incidence of the disorder is very low, 1 in 185 000, although it has a high frequency in some inbred populations.

The absence of affected members in other generations supports, but does not prove, autosomal recessive inheritance. The absence of consanguinity in this family allows the use of the general population incidence of the disorder to determine the risk of occurrence of MSUD in the woman's pregnancy.

Using the Hardy–Weinberg equilibrium, the carrier frequency for an autosomal recessive disorder can be derived from the disease incidence if it is known. Among non-inbred populations, the disease incidence of MSUD is 1 in 185 000.

$$p = \text{frequency of normal allele;}$$
$$q = \text{frequency of mutant allele}$$

$$q^2 = \text{disease incidence}$$
$$p + q = 1$$
$$p^2 + 2pq + q^2 = 1$$
$$2pq = \text{carrier frequency}$$
$$q^2 = 1/185,000$$
$$q = 1/430; \; p \text{ is approximately 1}$$

$2pq = 1$ in 215 (this is the chance that someone in the general population without a family history of the disorder will be a carrier for MSUD)

The woman's chance of being a carrier for MSUD is 1 in 215. Her husband is an obligate carrier because he has children affected by the condition. The risk of MSUD in the woman's pregnancy is 1 in 860 [1 (the chance that the husband is a carrier) $\times \; ^1/_2$ (the chance he transmits the mutation) $\times$ 1 in 215 (the chance that the wife is a carrier) $\times \; ^1/_2$ (the chance she transmits the mutant gene to their child)].

While the risk of MSUD in the woman's pregnancy is low, she is interested in whether prenatal diagnosis might be available.

Both OMIM and Genetests provide information about the molecular genetics of MSUD. Genetests provides information about the availability and sensitivity of molecular testing and other methods of carrier and disease detection.

MSUD is a genetically heterogeneous disorder. Mutations in three different genes have been recognized to cause the disorder with mutations in each gene accounting for about one-third of MSUD cases. In order to be affected, an individual must be homozygous or a compound heterozygote for mutations within the same gene. Individuals with two *MSUD* gene muta-

tions in different genes are not affected by MSUD. In contrast to cystic fibrosis and spinal muscular atrophy, where a common mutation accounts for the majority of gene carriers, individuals with MSUD all have uncommon mutations. Gene sequencing of the three *MSUD* genes will find about 95% of mutations in affected individuals.

The husband's children are not available for molecular testing. The husband is an obligate carrier of a MSUD gene mutation. He is willing to provide a blood sample.

Gene sequencing is laborious and expensive, especially when multiple genes must be examined. Before proceeding with molecular analysis, it is highly desirable to confirm the diagnosis of the affected child(ren) by review of their medical record(s) and to do gene sequencing on one of them first before testing other family members. If information about the affected child(ren)'s *MSUD* gene mutation status is not known, difficulties with interpretation of the father's results would arise if he were to carry a nucleotide variant of uncertain clinical importance or if he did not carry an identifiable sequence change in any of his *MSUD* genes.

The affected daughter's medical record becomes available for review and confirms her diagnosis of MSUD. Her father provides a blood sample for DNA testing. He has a mutation in the BCKA decarboxylase (E1) alpha subunit gene (BCKDHA gene).

The results have established the father's *MSUD* gene mutation. The father's second wife (the consultand) can then have gene sequencing of her *BCKDHA* gene. She does not need to have sequencing of her other two *MSUD* genes because mutations in those genes in combination with the husband's mutation will not cause MSUD in a child.

The a priori chance that the second wife is a carrier of a *BCKDHA* gene mutation is about 1 in 370 (starting with the assumption that the disease incidence of MSUD caused by *BCKDHA* gene mutations is one-third of the total MSUD incidence of 1 in 185 000, i.e., 1 in 555 000). If the wife does not have an identifiable mutation, her risk of being a *MSUD* gene carrier will have been reduced from 1 in 370 to 1 in 7400. The risk of an affected child would be 1 in 29 600 [1 (the chance the husband is a carrier) $\times \; ^1/_2$ (chance of transmission) $\times$ 1 in 7400 (the chance the wife is a carrier) $\times$ $^1/_2$ (the chance she transmits the abnormal gene to their child)]. Without an identifiable mutation in the wife, definitive prenatal diagnosis is not possible but the risk of an affected child is very small. In the unlikely event that the wife is a carrier of a *BCKDHA* gene mutation, the risk of MSUD in the pregnancy would be 25% and definitive prenatal diagnosis or preimplantation genetic diagnosis would be possible.

Further reading

1 Strauss KA, Puffenberger E, Morton DH (Updated January 2006). Maple Syrup Urine Disease. In: *GeneReviews* at GeneTests: Medical Genetics Information Resource (database online). Copyright, University of Washington, Seattle. 1997–2009. Available at http://www.genetests.org. Accessed September 2009.

X-Linked disorders

Features of X-linked inheritance

1 The trait is due to an abnormality of a gene on the X chromosome.
2 Male to male transmission does not occur.
3 All daughters of an affected male will inherit the abnormal gene.
4 Unaffected males do not transmit the abnormal gene to descendants of either sex; an exception is fragile X syndrome.
5 Each son of a carrier woman has a 50% chance of inheriting the trait.
6 Each daughter of a carrier woman has a 50% chance of being a carrier; for some X-linked diseases, females may manifest symptoms of variable severity.
7 For X-linked dominant disorders, each daughter and each son of a carrier woman has a 50% chance of being affected; there is often an excess of spontaneous abortions and stillbirths in males for X-linked dominant disorders.
8 Affected homozygous females are exceptional in X-linked disorders; they occur when an affected male and a carrier female have children.

Duchenne muscular dystrophy

Case 1 A woman requests genetic counseling in anticipation of a pregnancy. She is adopted and has just learned that she has two brothers with Duchenne muscular dystrophy who died in their late teens. Two other biological brothers are now in their 20s and unaffected. The brothers with muscular dystrophy were both diagnosed before age 5 years and were wheelchair-bound by age 12 years. A maternal uncle had Duchenne muscular dystrophy. Medical records are reviewed and show that the family participated in a research study two decades ago at the time the dystrophin gene was first identified. Abnormalities in this gene cause Duchenne muscular dystrophy. A deletion in the dystrophin gene was identified in the two affected brothers. A surprising finding in this family was the identification of the dystrophin gene deletion in one of her healthy biological brothers who is now in his 20s and has no medical problems. This brother declined to participate in further testing at the time of the research study. The females in the family were not tested in the research study.

Mutations in the *dystrophin* gene cause Duchenne muscular dystrophy, an X-linked disorder. Deletions of one or more exons of the *dystrophin* gene account for about 60% of disease-causing mutations. In our patient's situation, the presence of a familial *dystrophin* gene deletion means that there is no question about the accuracy of the clinical diagnosis. Our patient's mother is an obligate carrier of a *dystrophin* gene deletion because she had an affected brother and two affected sons. Thus, by pedigree analysis, our patient has a 50% risk of being a carrier. However, more information may be available about our patient that can be used to modify her risk.

Our patient reports that she has three sons and two daughters and is now in the first trimester of pregnancy. Her sons are 8, 10, and 12 years old and have no signs of Duchenne muscular dystrophy. The presence of three unaffected sons can be used in a Bayesian analysis to modify the risk that the patient carries the *dystrophin* gene deletion (Table 2.4).

The patient's risk of carrying the *dystrophin* gene deletion found in her affected brothers is $^1/_9$ (11%). If her fetus is male, his risk of having Duchenne muscular dystrophy is $^1/_{18}$ ($^1/_9 \times ^1/_2$) or about 6%.

Molecular analysis of the patient's DNA can determine whether she carries the *dystrophin* gene deletion. If she does, prenatal diagnosis by chorionic villus sampling or amniocentesis would be possible, as would preimplantation genetic diagnosis for a future pregnancy. Chorionic villus sampling is the preferred diagnostic procedure in this situation because it provides ample DNA without having to culture cells. Alternatively, women who wish to avoid an invasive procedure could have fetal sex determination at 16 weeks by ultrasonography and decline further testing if the fetus is female. Another option is the analysis of cell-free fetal DNA in maternal plasma by polymerase chain reaction assay to detect the fetal Y chromosome-associated *SRY* gene sequence. Although fetal DNA may be obtained as early as 5–7 weeks' gestation, laboratories may not offer this testing until 10–15 weeks' gestation. Ultrasonographic confirmation of a female fetus at 16 weeks' gestation would still be recommended.

Table 2.4 Risk for Duchenne muscular dystrophy (see case 1)

	Patient is a carrier	Patient is not a carrier
A priori risk	$^1/_2$	$^1/_2$
Three unaffected sons	$^1/_8$	1
Joint probability	$^1/_{16}$	$^1/_2$
Posterior probability	$\frac{1/16}{1/16 + 1/2} = 1/9$	$\frac{1/2}{1/2 + 1/16} = 8/9$

A phenotypic male with a *dystrophin* deletion should manifest classic symptoms of Duchenne muscular dystrophy. The patient questions why one of her brothers with the deletion has a normal phenotype. A sample or laboratory error or a coexisting chromosomal abnormality in the brother are possible explanations for the results of the brother's molecular testing. Presuming that the testing was repeated on the brother and the presence of the *dystrophin* deletion was confirmed, a peripheral blood karyotype followed by an array CGH study, if necessary, of the brother should be obtained.

The brother's peripheral blood karyotype is 47,XXY. He has Klinefelter syndrome.

The major features of Klinefelter syndrome include failure to develop male secondary sex characteristics at the time of puberty, gynecomastia, and infertility in the majority of affected individuals. There is also a chance of learning problems, mild motor difficulties such as poor coordination, shy personality, and tall stature. Most individuals with Klinefelter syndrome have an intelligence quotient that falls in the normal range but is usually 10–15 points below that of other siblings. However, some individuals with Klinefelter syndrome are only discovered during an evaluation for infertility, and some affected individuals may never be diagnosed at all.

With respect to X-linked disorders, a male with Klinefelter syndrome is functionally like a female because he has two X chromosomes. Females who are heterozygous for an X-linked disease very rarely have complete manifestations of the disorder because of the phenomenon of random X-chromosome inactivation which occurs in early embryogenesis. This results in gene expression from only one active X chromosome in each cell lineage. If the inactivation is random, half the cells will express the normal gene, which is sufficient to compensate for the cells expressing the abnormal gene. In this case, the brother with Klinefelter syndrome does not have manifestations of Duchenne muscular dystrophy because his normal *dystrophin* gene is active in a significant fraction of his cells.

Case 2 A woman is referred for genetic counseling early in her second pregnancy because she has a son with Duchenne muscular dystrophy secondary to a documented dystrophin gene deletion. A pedigree is collected; no other family members are affected. Molecular testing of the woman did not identify the dystrophin gene deletion.

Despite the absence of the *dystrophin* gene deletion in the DNA obtained from the woman's peripheral blood cells, there is still a significant risk of recurrence of Duchenne muscular dystrophy or a daughter who is a carrier. This is due to the high rate of germline mosaicism for *dystrophin* gene mutations. Empiric data show that this woman has a 10–15% chance of a recurrence of a child who carries the *dystrophin* gene deletion. Prenatal diagnosis for the *dystrophin* deletion should be offered to this woman; preimplantation genetic diagnosis is an option for future pregnancies.

Gonadal mosaicism plays an important role in the etiology of single gene disorders. Mosaicism can be restricted to the germ cells, somatic tissues, or both. Mosaicism may be clinically unimportant except for reproductive issues if restricted to the germline. If present in somatic tissues, clinical effects would range widely depending on the distribution and percentage of the abnormal cell line.

Gonadal mosaicism is more common for some disorders than for others. Relatively common genetic diseases in which there is a high frequency of gonadal mosaicism include Duchenne muscular dystrophy, tuberous sclerosis, and osteogenesis imperfecta type II in which there is a significant risk of recurrence in subsequent siblings. In contrast, gonadal mosaicism is rare among disorders caused by mutations in fibroblast growth factor receptor genes (e.g., achondroplasia, Apert syndrome). For many disorders, there is not enough published experience to estimate the chance of gonadal mosaicism.

Gonadal mosaicism for dominant disorders may complicate pedigree analysis where recurrences in siblings may lead to the erroneous conclusion of recessive inheritance.

This woman has a sister. What is the sister's chance of having a son with Duchenne muscular dystrophy?

The sister's risk of having a son affected by Duchenne muscular dystrophy is not increased above the background risk of about 1 in 5000. The *dystrophin* mutation arose as a postzygotic event in the woman.

Further reading

1 Bakker E, Veenema H, Den Dunnen JT *et al.* (1989) Germinal mosaicism increases the recurrence risk for "new" Duchenne muscular dystrophy mutations. *Journal of Medical Genetics* **26**(9):553–559.

2 Helderman-van den Enden AT, de Jong R *et al.* (2009) Recurrence risk due to germ line mosaicism: Duchenne and Becker muscular dystrophy *Clinical Genetics* **75** (5):465–472.

3 van Essen AJ, Abbs S, Baiget M *et al.* (1992) Parental origin and germline mosaicism of deletions and duplications of the dystrophin gene: a European study. *Human Genetics* **88**(3):249–257.

4 Zlotogora J (1998) Germ line mosaicism. *Human Genetics* **102**(4):381–386.

Hunter syndrome

A 24-year-old Hispanic woman and her husband seek genetic counseling because the woman has relatives with Hunter syndrome. She has two maternal aunts who have affected sons and another maternal aunt who has an affected grandson (Figure 2.3). The affected individuals died in their teens or early twenties; one is alive at age 3 years. The woman provides a photograph of an affected cousin which shows the classic facial appearance associated with the disorder. She wants genetic testing to establish whether she is at high risk for having an affected child. The woman's family is originally from a remote village in Central America where most of her family still lives.

Only males are affected in this family and they are all related to each other through their mothers or maternal grandmothers who are sisters. There is no evidence of male to male transmission. The family history is compatible with X-linked inheritance.

Because the woman is interested in genetic testing, it is crucial that the clinical diagnosis of Hunter syndrome that she reports in her affected cousins be confirmed by review of medical records. Although it is unlikely that the diagnosis of Hunter syndrome is incorrect based on the information we have collected thus far, the possibility of another disease with a similar presentation to Hunter syndrome cannot be excluded.

Hunter syndrome, also known as MPS II (mucopolysaccharidosis, type II) is an X-linked mucopolysaccharide storage disorder in which deficiency of the enzyme iduronate 2-sulfatase (IDS) causes multisystem abnormalities due to accumulation of glycosaminoglycans in body tissues. There is a wide range in age of onset, disease severity, and rate of progression of the disorder. Severe disease is associated with progressive cognitive deterioration and respiratory and cardiac disease leading to death in the first few decades of life. Associated findings include short stature, coarse facial features, macrocephaly with or without communicating hydrocephalus, macroglossia, hoarse voice, conductive and sensorineural hearing loss, hepatomegaly, splenomegaly, dysostosis multiplex, joint contractures, and spinal stenosis. The diagnosis of Hunter syndrome cannot be made definitively by clinical examination alone because other mucopolysaccaroidoses can have a similar presentation.

The severe form of another mucopolysaccharidosis, Hurler syndrome (MPS I), has a very similar clinical presentation to Hunter syndrome. Hurler syndrome has autosomal recessive inheritance. If the woman's family is extremely inbred with multiple consanguineous matings, the chance of a recessive condition mimicking the inheritance pattern of an X-linked disorder is increased. The patient's family is from an isolated village in Central America, increasing the likelihood of consanguineous

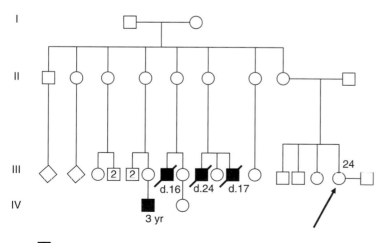

Figure 2.3 Pedigree of family with Hunter syndrome.

■ Hunter syndrome

matings, so it may be difficult to distinguish between autosomal recessive and X-linked recessive inheritance based on family history alone.

Before considering the possibility of carrier testing for our patient, confirmation of the diagnosis in one or more of her affected relatives by review of pertinent laboratory data is important. Diagnosis is made by finding deficient IDS enzyme activity in leukocytes, fibroblasts, or serum. If the clinical diagnosis is in error, carrier testing of our patient for Hunter syndrome would have no value.

> *Permission is granted by a maternal aunt who lives in the United States to review the medical records of her deceased affected son. Enzyme testing showed absent IDS in his plasma and massive excretion of glycosaminoglycans in his urine.*

The diagnosis of Hunter syndrome in this family is now confirmed. Carrier testing for our patient can now be considered. If laboratory results had not been available to confirm the diagnosis, mutation analysis of the *IDS* gene could have been undertaken but failure to find a disease-associated mutation would have left an unsatisfactory answer for the patient and for reproductive planning.

Pedigree analysis and application of Bayes' theorem are required to calculate the chance that our patient is a carrier of a mutation in her *IDS* gene, the only gene known to be associated with Hunter syndrome. Our patient's mother has three sisters (Figure 2.3, generation II) who are obligate carriers for an abnormal *IDS* gene. Since first-degree relatives share on average 50% of their genes, our patient's mother's a priori risk of being a carrier is 50%. However, our patient has two unaffected brothers, information that can be used to further refine her risk. Bayes' theorem allows us to calculate the probability that our patient's mother is a carrier given the conditional probability that she has two normal sons (Table 2.5).

Given that she has two normal sons, our patient's mother's revised risk of being a carrier of an abnormal *IDS* gene is 1 in 5. Our patient's risk of being a carrier is 1 in 10 (half of her mother's risk). The risk that our patient

would have an affected son is 1 in 40 [1 in 10 (chance that our patient is a carrier) $\times$ $^1/_2$ (chance that she transmits her abnormal *IDS* gene to the fetus) $\times$ $^1/_2$ (chance that the fetus is male)]. Based on this information, the patient wants to know whether she is a carrier for Hunter syndrome.

Measurement of IDS activity in serum or white blood cells is not reliable for detection of carrier females as a carrier may have normal enzyme activity resulting from the vagaries of X-chromosome inactivation. Molecular analysis to establish the presence or absence of a disease-causing mutation in our patient is the only approach to accurate carrier detection.

Only one gene, *IDS*, is known to be associated with Hunter syndrome. DNA-based carrier testing can be accomplished for our patient if gene sequencing identifies the disease-causing mutation in an affected family member. A negative (normal) gene sequencing result in a woman is only a true negative result if a disease-causing mutation in an affected family member has been documented. In a small number of families, the disease-causing mutation cannot be detected by current testing methods. Furthermore, partial deletions in the *IDS* gene account for about 10% of mutations; partial gene deletions are technically more difficult to find in females than in males.

> *The patient has an affected living first cousin once removed (Figure 2.3, generation IV). Obtaining a blood sample from him for IDS gene testing is indicated, but he lives in a remote village in Central America and is not available for testing.*

There are no other living affected males in the patient's family. However, she has three maternal aunts who are obligate carriers of a mutation in their *IDS* gene. Analysis of DNA from one of the aunts has a high probability of providing useful information.

> *The patient has one maternal aunt who lives in the United States. However, she is fearful of needles and refuses to give a blood sample.*

Many laboratories are willing to extract DNA from buccal cells or saliva samples. The molecular diagnostics laboratory is willing to accept a saliva sample from the maternal aunt.

> *Gene sequencing of the maternal aunt's IDS genes identified one copy of a nucleotide change in exon 4 of the IDS gene. The nucleotide change is predicted to result in a tryptophan to serine change at amino acid position 153 in the IDS protein.*

Table 2.5 Risk for Hunter syndrome (see case)

	Patient's mother is a carrier	Patient's mother is not a carrier
A priori risk	$^1/_2$	$^1/_2$
Two unaffected sons	$^1/_4$	1
Joint probability	$^1/_8$	$^1/_2$
Posterior probability	$\frac{1/8}{1/8+1/2} = 1/5$	$\frac{1/2}{1/2+1/8} = 4/5$

It is now important to establish whether this nucleotide change is a deleterious mutation or a benign sequence polymorphism. There are a number of criteria that can be used to assess whether a gene sequence change is disease-causing:

1 Is it a previously documented silent polymorphism or pathogenic mutation? There are constantly updated databases that would have this information.

2 Does the nucleotide change segregate with the disease in the family?

3 What are the predicted and demonstrated effects on the protein or RNA product?

4 What is the extent of evolutionary conservation of the affected nucleotide or protein?

Review of the National Center for Biotechnology Information database indicates that the nucleotide change found in our patient's maternal aunt has not been previously reported in patients with Hunter syndrome. In this family, it has not been documented in an affected family member or other obligate carrier females.

The nucleotide change results in a tryptophan to serine change at amino acid position 153. These two amino acids have very different chemical properties, which could have a dramatic effect on protein structure and function.

This amino acid is conserved in humans, a variety of other mammals, and some invertebrates.

The effects on protein structure and the high conservation of the amino acid suggest that the nucleotide change is pathogenic although caution about this conclusion is still warranted.

Documentation of the nucleotide change in an affected family member and in other obligate carrier females in the family would strengthen the conclusion that it is pathogenic. Documentation that the nucleotide change is absent in the patient's unaffected maternal uncles and in the patient's unaffected brothers would provide further support for its pathogenicity.

The patient travels to Central America to obtain a saliva sample on her affected cousin once removed (individual IV-1). Analysis of DNA obtained from his saliva documents the presence of the nucleotide change. The patient cannot afford to test other family members.

The nucleotide change has now been documented in two family members providing further support, but not conclusive evidence, that it segregates with the disease.

The patient provides a blood sample for carrier testing herself. Analysis of her DNA indicates the presence of the nucleotide change.

The patient is counseled that she is a carrier of this variant in the *IDS* gene and the mutation is very likely to be pathogenic. Her risk of being a carrier for Hunter syndrome likely approaches 100%. The patient is offered the option of preimplantation genetic diagnosis and prenatal diagnosis for the *IDS* gene nucleotide change. The patient becomes pregnant without having preimplantation genetic diagnosis.

If the patient has a son, the risk of Hunter syndrome approaches 50%, and she wants information as early in the pregnancy as possible. Chorionic villus sampling is the preferable procedure in this situation because a large amount of DNA can be obtained and analyzed quickly without having to culture cells. Alternatively, if a woman wanted to avoid invasive testing, ultrasonographic examination could be performed at 15 weeks' gestation and amniocentesis performed only if the fetus were male.

Because there is still not complete confidence that the patient's *IDS* gene nucleotide change is disease-causing, another independent method of prenatal diagnosis would be ideal. In this situation, enzyme based testing of chorionic villus cells is also recommended. Unfortunately, prenatal diagnosis of Hunter syndrome by enzyme-based testing is only available at an overseas laboratory and the patient cannot afford the high expense.

Chorionic villus sampling is performed at 11 weeks' gestation. The chorionic villus cell karyotype is 46,XY. Analysis of DNA obtained from uncultured chorionic villi indicates that the fetus has inherited the IDS *gene nucleotide change found in his mother and affected cousin. The patient elects pregnancy termination. Biochemical analysis of fetal skin fibroblasts obtained after pregnancy termination shows negligible activity of IDS, confirming unequivocally that the fetus was affected by Hunter syndrome and providing further evidence that the nucleotide change found in the woman's* IDS *gene is pathogenic.*

Further reading

1 Froissart R, Da Silva IM, Maire I (2007) Mucopolysaccharidosis type II: an update on mutation spectrum. *Acta Paediatrica Supplement* **96**(455):71–77.

2 Froissart R, Moreira da Silva I, Guffon N (2002) Mucopolysaccharidosis type II – genotype/phenotype aspects. *Acta Paediatrica Supplement* **91**(439):82–87.

3 Martin RA (Updated 11/6/2007). Mucopolysaccharidosis type II. In: *GeneReviews* at GeneTests: Medical Genetics Information Resource (database online). Copyright, University of Washington, Seattle. 1997–2009. Available at http://www.genetests.org. Accessed September 2009.

4 Martin R, Beck M, Eng C *et al.* (2008) Recognition and diagnosis of mucopolysaccharidosis II (Hunter syndrome). *Pediatrics* **121**(2):e377–386.

5 Wraith JE, Scarpa M, Beck M *et al.* (2008) Mucopolysaccharidosis type II (Hunter syndrome): a clinical review and recommendations for treatment in the era of enzyme replacement therapy. *European Journal of Pediatrics* **167**(3):267–277.

Fragile X syndrome

Case 1 A 33-year-old primiparous woman is referred for urgent consultation at 22 weeks' gestation because she was just diagnosed as a fragile X syndrome gene carrier following the diagnosis of fragile X syndrome in her first cousin (her father's sister's son) who has autistic spectrum disorder and mental retardation. Ultrasonographic examination indicates that she is carrying a male fetus. The woman's family history includes a sister who had premature menopause at age 38 years and her father, age 72, who was recently diagnosed with Parkinson disease. Further information is collected and reveals that the woman's father has another brother whose daughter's son has autistic spectrum disorder.

Fragile X syndrome is an X-linked trinucleotide repeat disorder which is caused by large expansions of a CGG nucleotide triplet repeat in the *FMR1* gene. The normal gene has less than 45 repeats. All males with a full *FMR1* gene mutation (CGG expansions of ≥200 repeats) have moderate to severe mental retardation and about half of females with a full mutation have mild mental retardation or learning disabilities. Autistic spectrum disorder is a commonly associated finding. CGG expansions of 55–199 repeats are termed premutations. In females, CGG triplet repeats of 55–199 are unstable and are prone to large expansions during meiosis. The risk of expansion to a full mutation is correlated with the size of the premutation as shown in Table 2.6. Premutations in males may change upon transmission to offspring but almost never expand into the full mutation range. CGG triplet repeat sizes between 45 and 54 may occasionally be unstable during meiosis but are not susceptible to large expansions in a single generation. In the literature, the smallest number of

Table 2.6 Risk of fragile X syndrome in offspring based on maternal FMR1 gene premutation size

# Maternal CGG repeats	Chance of expansion to a full mutation	Chance of son affected by fragile X syndrome	Chance of daughter affected by fragile X syndrome
56–59	3.7%	1–2%	0.5–1%
60–69	5.3%	2–3%	1–2%
70–79	31.1%	15%	7%
80–89	57.8%	30%	15%
90–99	80.1%	40%	20%
>100	~100%	50%	25%

Adapted from Nolin SL Brown WT, Glicksman A *et al.* (2003) *American Journal of Human Genetics* **72**:454–464.

repeats that has expanded to a full mutation has been 56 repeats.

The risk of fragile X syndrome in our patient's fetus depends on the number of CGG repeats in her abnormal *FMR1* gene.

Molecular analysis of our patient's FMR1 *genes shows repeat sizes of 37 and 105 CGG repeats.*

As shown in Table 2.6, if the patient has transmitted her abnormal *FMR1* gene to the fetus, risk of expansion to a full mutation in this and future pregnancies is 100%. Thus, the risk of fragile X syndrome in the current pregnancy is 50% because the patient could also have transmitted her normal-sized *FMR1* gene. Analysis of DNA obtained from amniotic fluid cells or chorionic villi can establish the *FMR1* gene status of the fetus. Preimplantation genetic diagnosis is also available for future pregnancies.

If a fetus is female and inherits an FMR1 *gene full mutation, can definitive predictions about phenotypic effects be made?*

About half of females with an FMR1 gene mutation have mild mental retardation or learning disabilities. Predictions cannot be made prenatally.

The patient's family history also illustrates other important features of *FMR1* gene mutations. For almost all X-linked disorders which have major manifestations in the first few years of life, an unaffected adult male may be excluded as transmitting the abnormal gene to an affected child. In fragile X syndrome, however, the abnormal *FMR1* gene can be transmitted by both unaffected females as well as unaffected males. Unaffected males with *FMR1* gene premutations will transmit their premutation to each of their daughters, who in turn are at increased risk for having children with full mutations. Thus, pedigrees of families with fragile X syndrome show unaffected obligate carrier males transmitting an abnormal gene which manifests as disease in their grandchildren or subsequent generations.

Another unique feature of this trinucleotide repeat disorder is the association of abnormal triplet repeat sizes with other pathology in addition to the classic expression of fragile X syndrome. Premature ovarian failure, at age 40 or less, occurs in about 20% of women who carry a fragile X premutation but not in those who carry a full mutation. The diagnosis of premature ovarian failure is an indication for fragile X syndrome carrier testing, especially if a woman is considering assisted reproductive technology using her own ova. A woman might go through expensive fertility treatments unaware that she is at high risk for having a child with fragile X syndrome. The incidence of *FMR1* gene premutations in women with premature ovarian failure is about 14%.

Another exceptional characteristic of fragile X syndrome is the association of *FMR1* gene premutations with fragile X tremor and ataxia syndrome (FXTAS), a neurodegenerative disorder associated with progressive cognitive impairment and cerebellar ataxia. For males over 50 years of age, the overall prevalence of FXTAS is 40%. By age 80 years, 75% of premutation carrier males will have signs of FXTAS. The incidence of *FMR1* premutations in males with an adult-onset cerebellar ataxia who have no other similarly affected relatives is about 3%. Female premutation carriers are only occasionally affected by FXTAS.

Recognition of the protean manifestations of *FMR1* gene mutations allows for identification of relatives at high risk for having children with fragile X syndrome. Furthermore, the diagnosis of fragile X syndrome in a child increases the risk of premature ovarian failure and FXTAS in other relatives. Alerting other relatives to this increased risk will hopefully result in more focused, less invasive and less expensive diagnostic evaluations should symptoms develop.

Further reading

1 Berry-Kravis E, Abrams L, Coffey SM *et al.* (2007) Fragile X-associated tremor/ataxia syndrome: clinical features, genetics, and testing guidelines. *Movement Disorders* **22**:14:2018–2030.

2 Bretherick KL, Fluker MR, Robinson WP (2005) FMR1 repeat sizes in the gray zone and high end of the normal range are associated with premature ovarian failure. *Human Genetics* **117**(4): 376–382.

3 Brussino A, Gellera C, Saluto A *et al.* (2005) A. FMR1 gene premutation is a frequent genetic cause of late-onset sporadic cerebellar ataxia. *Neurology* **64**(1): 145–147.

4 Fernandez-Carvajal I, Posadas BL, Pan R *et al.* (2009) Expansion of an *FMR1* grey-zone allele to a full mutation in two generations. *Journal of Molecular Diagnostics* **11**(4):306–309.

5 Nolin SL, Brown WT, Glicksman A *et al.* (2003) Expansion of the fragile X CGG repeat in females with premutation or intermediate alleles. *American Journal of Human Genetics* **72**:454–464.

Factor VIII deficiency (hemophilia A)

A woman is referred for genetic counseling early in her first pregnancy. She was incidentally diagnosed at 4 months of age with severe hemophilia A (factor VIII deficiency) during her preoperative evaluation for repair of an inguinal hernia. Her factor VIII activity is less than 1%. She has required treatment with recombinant factor VIII after minor trauma. She has had a few episodes of spontaneous intra-articular bleeding. She has a maternal uncle and younger brother with severe hemophilia (factor VIII activity levels less than 1%). Her mother and father have normal factor VIII activity. The woman is concerned about having a child with severe hemophilia.

Hemophilia A or factor VIII deficiency is caused by mutations in the factor VIII gene on the X chromosome. The severe form of the disorder results in a serious bleeding diathesis in affected males who have only one X chromosome. In females, inactivation of one of the two X chromosomes occurs very early in embryogenesis, resulting in the situation where genes on only one of their two X chromosomes are expressed in each somatic cell. Thus, females who are heterozygous for an X-linked mutant gene have on average about half of their cells containing an X chromosome with the normal gene expressed, which in the case of factor VIII deficiency is usually sufficient for normal hemostasis.

Why would a female have classic manifestations of an X-linked disorder? This phenomenon occurs rarely and may be explained by a number of different mechanisms.

Cytogenetic abnormalities involving a reciprocal translocation between one of the X chromosomes and an autosome results in non-random X-inactivation. The X chromosome which possesses autosomal material is active in all viable cells. Thus, if the X chromosome involved in the translocation bears the mutant gene, that gene will be expressed in all of a woman's cells and she will be functionally like a male with respect to expression of an X-linked disease. Other chromosomal abnormalities such as Turner syndrome, Turner syndrome variants, and X chromosome deletions with a mutation on the intact X chromosome may occur. Thus, in any female manifesting classic symptoms of an X-linked disorder, a metaphase karyotype of peripheral blood cells is indicated. Array comparative genomic hybridization (CGH) could also be performed to look for small X chromosome deletions. Current array CGH techniques would not detect a balanced X;autosome translocation but molecular methods under development will likely be available in the near future. If the peripheral blood karyotype is normal and a Turner syndrome variant is suspected based on other clinical findings, fluorescent in situ hybridization (FISH) analysis of another tissue (e.g., buccal cells) as well as on a large number of interphase blood cells could be performed to look for the presence of an abnormal cell line.

Because one of two X chromosomes is randomly inactivated in early embryogenesis, cells with the maternally and paternally derived active X chromosomes should, on average, be present in equal amounts in the tissues of a female. However, because the process of X-chromosome inactivation is a random event, the distribution of maternally and paternally derived X chromosomes in a population of women follows a normal or Gaussian distribution curve. Thus, by chance alone, there may be significant distortions in the distribution of cells with maternally or paternally active X chromosomes, resulting in certain tissues having a preponderance of cells with the active X chromosome that bears a mutation.

For some X-linked immunodeficiency disorders, cells in hematopoietic lineages with the active X chromosome bearing the disease-causing mutation are at a survival disadvantage in carrier females. This results in a pattern of X-chromosome inactivation in surviving cells that is skewed in favor of the X chromosome that bears the normal allele.

Mutations in the *XIST* gene, the gene which controls X-inactivation, or other genes involved in the X-chromosome inactivation process, have also been postulated as an explanation for skewed X-chromosome inactivation. Support for this hypothesis comes from families in which several generations of women demonstrate only a paternally derived active X chromosome. The pattern of transmission in these families is consistent with X-linked dominant inheritance. In these rare families, defects in the X-inactivation process itself result in selective inactivation of the maternal X chromosome. Thus, if the father has an X-linked disease himself or if a de novo disease-causing mutation on his X chromosome arose in his sperm which conceived a daughter, she would be expected to manifest classic symptoms of the disorder.

Other unlikely scenarios which could explain the severe manifestations of an X-linked disease in a female include inheritance of her mother's factor VIII gene mutation and a paternally derived de novo mutation in the factor VIII gene that occurred in the father's sperm. Uniparental isodisomy for the maternal X chromosome would be another explanation for a female who displays severe symptoms of an X-linked disorder.

A metaphase karyotype is obtained on the affected woman. Cytogenetic studies reveal a reciprocal translocation of part of the long arm of an X chromosome and part of the short arm of a chromosome 5. Molecular studies using DNA polymorphisms show that the two chromosomes involved in the translocation are maternally derived.

In X;autosome translocations, there may be non-random X-inactivation or cell death if the X chromosome with the autosomal material is inactivated. The genes on the autosomal segment of the translocation must be expressed. In this woman's situation, her paternally inherited X chromosome with the normal factor VIII gene is not active, rendering her the equivalent of a male with respect to disease expression due to an X-linked gene inherited from her mother.

The translocation in this woman almost certainly arose as a de novo event. Her mother has a normal blood cell karyotype (see Figure 2.4). Also, her mother, who is an obligate carrier of the factor VIII gene mutation, has normal factor VIII activity, which is evidence that she does not have skewed X inactivation.

Women who carry X;autosome translocations may have reduced fertility, especially if the translocation breakpoint on the X chromosome involves regions of the X chromosome (Xq13 and q27) which are associated with premature ovarian failure. In a fertile woman with an X;autosome translocation, about half of her gametes will have various combinations of unbalanced chromosomes, resulting in a significant risk for chromosomally unbalanced conceptuses, some of which may be viable in the second trimester or after birth. Males with an X;autosome

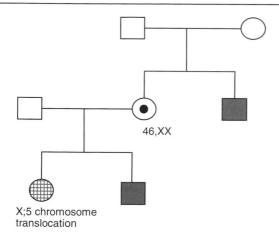

46,XX

X;5 chromosome
translocation

■ Severe factor VIII deficiency
⊕ Severe factor VIII deficiency and chromosome X;5 translocation
□ ○ Normal factor VIII activity
⊙ Carrier of gene for severe factor VIII deficiency who has
normal factor VIII activity

Figure 2.4 Pedigree of family with factor VIII deficiency.

translocation may be phenotypically normal or may have genital defects; all are likely to be infertile. Females with balanced X;autosome translocations would most likely have the same phenotype as their mother, which in this woman's situation would predict that any daughter with the balanced translocation would be affected by severe factor VIII deficiency.

Prenatal diagnosis with chromosome analysis will identify embryos which have unbalanced chromosomes or the chromosomal translocation. Sequencing of the woman's hemophilia gene could identify the factor VIII mutation which could be used for preimplantation and prenatal genetic diagnosis for hemophilia A.

Obstetric management of a woman with severe hemophilia presents unique medical challenges which are not addressed in this discussion. If this woman can successfully conceive, published reports show that careful multidisciplinary planning and use of recombinant factor VIII concentrates will enable a good outcome.

Further reading

1 Leuer M, Oldenburg J, Lavergne JM *et al.* (2001) Somatic mosaicism in hemophilia A: a fairly common event. *American Journal of Human Genetics* **69**(1):75–87.
2 Puck JM, Willard HF (1998) X Inactivation in females with X-linked disease. *New England Journal of Medicine* **338**(5):325–328.
3 Pavlova A, Brondke H, Müsebeck J *et al.* (2009) Molecular mechanisms underlying hemophilia A phenotype in seven females. *Journal of Thrombosis and Haemostasis* **7**(6):976–982.
4 Oldenburg J, Ananyeva NM, Saenko EL (2004) Molecular basis of haemophilia. *Haemophilia* **10**:Suppl 4:133–139.

X-linked adrenoleukodystrophy

A 22-year-old woman who is a late registrant for prenatal care is referred for genetic counseling because her partner has a first cousin with spina bifida. Upon collection of the woman's family history, it was disclosed that her father died at age 47 years of a neurodegenerative disorder. Review of the father's hospital record showed that he was well until his mid 40s when he developed memory loss, confusion, difficulty with reading and writing, visual impairment, and emotional lability followed by rapid neurologic deterioration and death. A CT scan revealed diffuse white matter disease. Biochemical analysis of his plasma showed marked elevations of very long chain fatty acids (VLCFA) and an increased ratio of VLCFA to long chain fatty acids, a diagnostic hallmark of X-linked adrenoleukodystrophy. At the time of his diagnosis, his wife (the consultand's mother) received genetic counseling about the genetic implications of the disorder for the couple's children and other relatives. The consultand has two sisters, a brother, and two paternal aunts. The family history also includes one paternal uncle of the consultand who died at age 43 years following a 10-year psychiatric hospitalization, raising the possibility that he too was affected by adrenoleukodystrophy.

While the woman can be reassured that she is at low risk of occurrence of a child with a neural tube defect, she is at high risk for having children with a devastating genetic disease. The woman is informed that, based on her father's diagnosis, she is an obligate carrier for X-linked adrenoleukodystrophy. If her fetus is male, he has a 50% chance of developing the disorder. Because the woman's father first showed symptoms of adrenoleukodystrophy in his 40s, the woman states that she is unconcerned because she believes that effective treatment of the disorder will be available by the time an affected son would reach adulthood.

X-linked adrenoleukodystrophy, an inflammatory demyelinating disorder affecting the central nervous system white matter including the spinal cord and adrenal glands, has striking and highly variable phenotypic expression and is the most common of the peroxisomal disorders. It is caused by mutations in the *ABCD1* gene located on the long arm of the X chromosome and has an incidence of about 1 in 20 000 males with no ethnic predilection. The biochemical hallmark is elevated plasma and tissue levels of VLCFA due to reduced beta-oxidation of VLCFA in peroxisomes. Peroxisomes are cellular organelles that are involved in cellular functions including the metabolism of VLCFA by beta-oxidation, production of plasmalogen, synthesis of bile acid, and the breakdown of peroxides.

The adult-onset form of adrenoleukodystrophy, known as adrenomyeloneuropathy, accounts for slightly less than half of cases and usually has onset in the third to fifth decades. Adrenomyeloneuropathy can be rapidly progressive with cerebral involvement as seen in this woman's father, or can progress slowly over several decades with primarily spinal cord involvement causing progressive stiffness, weakness in the lower extremities, abnormalities of sphincter control, sexual dysfunction, and in a subset of men, rapid neurologic deterioration at the end of life. About 30% of affected males have the childhood cerebral form with onset usually between ages 3 and 10 years, in which a variable period of totally normal development is followed by progressive neurologic deterioration resulting in total disability, with death ensuing after a few years. Five to 10% of affected boys develop the severe childhood cerebral form in their teens. Adrenal insufficiency as the only manifestation of the disorder is common in younger ages but most of these individuals will eventually develop the severe childhood form or adrenomyeloneuropathy. Even among affected male relatives within the same family, the phenotypes are often diverse.

As expected from the highly variable expression of disease among members of the same family, there is no correlation between the underlying mutation in the *ABCD1* gene and the severity and age of onset of symptoms. Other unidentified epigenetic factors may play a role in the variability of disease expression. Treatment of adrenoleukodystrophy includes adrenal hormone replacement therapy for adrenal insufficiency but this does not ameliorate the progressive neurologic course of the disease. Allogeneic stem cell or bone marrow transplantation has been successful in delaying or preventing the onset of symptoms in affected boys who have not yet shown signs of significant neurodegeneration but who have white matter abnormalities on MRI.

The efficacy of dietary treatments, including the use of a mixture of erucic and oleic acids ("Lorenzo's oil") to normalize VLCFA levels in plasma and tissues, is also under investigation.

The woman decides that she wants prenatal diagnosis of adrenoleukodystrophy.

Ultrasonographic examination is indicated to establish the fetal gender. If the fetus is female, the risk of severe disease in childhood is very small. Among female heterozygotes, about half have mild sensory changes in their lower extremities in adulthood, several percent develop adrenomyeloneuropathy, and a few percent have cerebral involvement. The presence of symptoms in a significant fraction of adult carrier females shows that the normal *ABCD1* gene does not completely compensate for the abnormal allele in the presence of random X-inactivation.

The fetus appears to be male by ultrasonographic examination. Amniocentesis is performed and the fetus is a chromosomally normal male who has markedly elevated concentrations of VLCFA and a high ratio of VLCFA to long chain fatty acids in cultured amniocytes. The fetus is affected with adrenoleukodystrophy.

The woman is given the option of pregnancy termination. Unfortunately, predictions about when symptoms of adrenoleukodystrophy will present themselves cannot be made prenatally or after delivery. There is a significant chance that the baby would have onset of cerebral symptoms during the first decade of life despite the later age of onset seen in the woman's father. After delivery, the baby needs to be monitored closely by pediatric specialists for signs of adrenal insufficiency and early signs of neurologic disease. Experimental treatments can be considered. If the pregnancy continues, the results of prenatal diagnosis should be confirmed after delivery by analysis of plasma concentrations of VLCFA.

With respect to future pregnancies for the woman, prenatal diagnosis can be accomplished earlier by measurement of VLCFA in chorionic villi. Sequencing of the *ABCD1* gene can find 98% of disease-causing mutations in affected individuals. Prenatal diagnosis by molecular analysis would also be possible if the disease-causing mutation in the woman's family is identified. It would also give the woman the option for preimplantation genetic diagnosis.

The woman was unaware of the genetic implications of her father's diagnosis despite evidence in the medical record of extensive discussions and written communication with the woman's mother by the physicians involved in the father's diagnosis. This might be due to poor comprehension or denial on the part of the woman's mother, the woman herself, or a misguided effort by the woman's mother to protect her children from difficult information. The woman has two sisters who are also obligate carriers for adrenoleukodystrophy and are at risk for having affected sons; they need to be made aware of the availability of preimplantation genetic diagnosis and prenatal testing. Other female relatives of the father, such as his two sisters, are also at significant risk for being carriers. It is important that genetic counseling of the woman includes an offer to counsel other members of the family. Provision of written information can facilitate the transmission of accurate information to other family members. In addition to the reproductive issues for heterozygous women, they face an increased risk of developing neurologic problems related to adrenoleukodystrophy as they age. Knowledge of a woman's adrenoleukodystrophy carrier status can help guide a diagnostic evaluation and hopefully spare a symptomatic woman unnecessary diagnostic procedures or ineffective treatments.

Further reading

1 Moser AB, Steinberg SJ, Raymong GV (Updated 6/2/2009). X-linked Adrenoleukodystrophy. In: *GeneReviews* at GeneTests: Medical Genetics Information Resource (database online). Copyright, University of Washington, Seattle. 1997–2009. Available at http://www.genetests.org. Accessed September 2009.

2 Moser HW, Mahmood A, Raymond GV (2007) X-linked adrenoleukodystrophy. *Nature Clinical Practice, Neurology* **3**(3):140–151.

3 Moser HW, Loes DJ, Melhem ER *et al.* (2000) X-Linked adrenoleukodystrophy: overview and prognosis as a function of age and brain magnetic resonance imaging abnormality. A study involving 372 patients. *Neuropediatrics* **31**(5):227–239.

4 Moser AB, Moser HW (1999) The prenatal diagnosis of X-linked adrenoleukodystrophy. *Prenatal Diagnosis* **19**:46–48.

Skeletal dysplasias

Skeletal dysplasias, as a class of birth defects, are one of the more common entities that are diagnosable by prenatal ultrasonographic examination. They are included in this chapter on Mendelian inheritance because virtually all of the skeletal dysplasias are due to single gene defects. There are more than 200 different skeletal dysplasias, defined as disorders associated with disturbances of growth of bone or cartilage. They are associated with varying degrees of abnormalities in the shape, size, texture, and proportion of the limbs, trunk, and skull. Clinical expression ranges from disorders which are lethal in utero or in the perinatal period to conditions that are unassociated with significant morbidity postnatally. The likelihood of in utero identification by ultrasonographic examination is highly correlated with the severity of the disorder. However, the precise diagnosis of a skeletal dysplasia is often difficult to make by prenatal ultrasonographic examination because of the large number of possible diagnostic entities which have overlapping and variable features.

While the molecular basis of the common skeletal dysplasias is largely understood, the underlying genetic defects causing many of the rare disorders remain unknown. Many skeletal dysplasias, especially those which are severe, arise de novo due to new dominant mutations, and are discovered during routine sonography in the second or third trimester. When severe abnormalities are present, prognosis can be made based on the nature of the abnormalities alone. For example, a small thorax may be associated with hypoplastic lungs. Early and severe shortening, bowing and/or multiple fractures of the long bones with marked hypomineralization of the skull, are markers of severe skeletal dysplasias which are usually lethal in the newborn period.

Identification of the underlying molecular basis is sometimes possible via amniocentesis or placental biopsy if the ultrasonographic findings are strongly suggestive of a specific diagnosis. Often, however, pathologic examination and biochemical and imaging studies performed postnatally are required to narrow the differential diagnosis and direct the approach to molecular testing. Elucidating the underlying molecular or biochemical defect, while not always possible despite extensive evaluation, allows for accurate counseling about recurrence risks and provides the opportunity for earlier prenatal diagnosis in future pregnancies. For some severe skeletal dysplasias, ultrasonographic examination beginning early in the second trimester will find most affected fetuses.

This section illustrates the challenges in counseling posed by the genetic heterogeneity of some of the autosomal recessive skeletal dysplasias for which gene-based diagnosis is not yet available. In addition, gonadal mosaicism is another recurring theme in the genetics of some of the skeletal dysplasias. For disorders compatible with long-term survival, assortative mating among affected individuals, who both have short stature, increases the risk for offspring who are double heterozygotes for two different skeletal dysplasias, or are homozygotes or compound heterozygotes for a single gene disorder that is usually seen in the heterozygous form. These situations pose major challenges in counseling about prognosis.

Achondroplasia and hypochondroplasia

A couple is referred for genetic counseling because they have the typical findings of achondroplasia with disproportionately short arms and legs, frontal bossing, and midface hypoplasia. The wife is 3'9" tall and the husband is 4'4" tall. The wife's surgical history is significant for an L2-L3 laminectomy/discectomy, an osteotomy, and multiple myringotomies. She is 36 years old and was diagnosed in the newborn period. Her husband is 38 years old and has an unremarkable medical history. His frontal bossing is less pronounced than that seen in his wife and, surprisingly, he was not diagnosed with achondroplasia until almost 3 years of age. Both report that their siblings and parents have normal stature. The couple would like to have children and want information about the chance that a child would have a more severe form of achondroplasia than they manifest.

Dominant heterozygous mutations in the fibroblast growth factor receptor 3 (*FGFR3*) gene are the cause of achondroplasia, with a single G-to-A point mutation at nucleotide 1138 of the *FGFR3* gene accounting for 98% of cases. One to two percent of affected individuals have another point mutation or an uncharacterized mutation. About 80% of cases arise de novo. Achondroplasia is the most common skeletal dysplasia.

When both members of the couple have achondroplasia, the chance in each pregnancy that a baby will be heterozygous, like both parents, is 50%. There is a 25% chance in each pregnancy that the child will be of normal stature and a 25% chance in each pregnancy that the fetus will inherit both parents' *FGFR3* mutations. This latter situation, homozygosity for the *FGFR3* mutation, is usually a lethal condition in early infancy due to respiratory compromise caused by chest size constriction and neurologic problems associated with hydrocephalus.

The couple indicates that they would pursue prenatal diagnosis of homozygous achondroplasia in a future pregnancy. They state that they would be accepting of a child with a similar skeletal dysplasia to themselves or a child with normal stature.

In order for chorionic villus sampling or preimplantation genetic diagnosis to be accomplished, the *FGFR3* mutations in both parents need to be identified. It should not be assumed that both parents carry the common *FGFR3* mutation associated with achondroplasia, and there is a chance, albeit small, that one (or both) of the parents has another skeletal dysplasia with a different molecular basis that clinically resembles achondroplasia. This latter possibility is increased in this case because the husband's diagnosis of achondroplasia at age 3 years is atypical. Without knowledge of the parents' *FGFR* mutations, results of chorionic villus sampling predicting a heterozygous or homozygous unaffected fetus could be in error and would not allow definitive predictions about the achondroplasia status of the fetus.

Ultrasonographic examination also has utility in the prenatal diagnosis of both heterozygous and homozygous achondroplasia. However, the skeletal findings of homozygous achondroplasia are usually not apparent until 18–20 weeks' gestation. The sonographic findings of heterozygous achondroplasia usually become evident in the late second trimester or early third trimester.

The couple elects testing of their FGFR3 *genes. The wife, as expected, is heterozygous for the G-to-A point mutation at nucleotide 1138 of the* FGFR3 *gene, the most common mutation associated with achondroplasia. However, gene sequencing of the husband's* FGFR3 *genes does not identify a mutation. He is examined by a clinical geneticist who believes that he has hypochondroplasia which has a similar, but milder, presentation than achondroplasia.*

Hypochondroplasia is heterogeneous and in most reported cases associated with specific *FGFR3* gene mutations that are different from the ones causing achondroplasia. Some individuals, like the husband, who meet the diagnostic criteria for hypochondroplasia do not have detectable mutations in the *FGFR3* genes. It is uncertain whether these individuals have *FGFR3* mutations that cannot be detected by current testing methods or whether they have mutations at another chromosomal locus.

If the father has an undetectable mutation in the *FGFR3* gene then the risk of a heterozygous affected fetus is 50%. There is a 25% risk of a compound heterozygote (two different alleles at a single specific locus) and a 25% chance of an unaffected fetus. If the father has a dominant mutation at a different genetic locus, there would be a 25% chance of double heterozygosity (two different alleles at two different loci). Again, the risk of inheriting the maternal *FGFR3* mutation would be 50%, and the chance of an unaffected fetus would be 25%. Without molecular identification of the mutation causing the husband's skeletal dysplasia, definitive prenatal diagnosis of a fetus who is a compound heterozygote or double heterozygote for both parents' mutations is not possible. Furthermore, information is now needed about the clinical presentation of a fetus who is a compound heterozygote or double heterozygote.

Homozygosity for *FGFR3* mutations causing achondroplasia is almost always a lethal condition with death occurring in the newborn period or later in infancy. Compound heterozygosity for mutations causing achondroplasia and hypochondroplasia is also a severe condition but is not uniformly lethal. Long-term survival with severe skeletal abnormalities, moderate restrictive lung disease, developmental delay, mental retardation, and seizures has been reported.

The couple is highly motivated to have a child unaffected by compound heterozygosity or double heterozygosity for achondroplasia/hypochondroplasia.

If the fetus did not inherit the wife's *FGFR3* gene mutation, the fetus could be confidently predicted to be unaffected by compound or double heterozygosity. The chance of hypochondroplasia, with a phenotype similar to the father's, would be 50%. However, if the fetus inherited the wife's *FGFR3* gene mutation, the risk of compound or double heterozygosity for achondroplasia/hypochondroplasia would be 50% and no further early diagnostic testing would be available. Waiting for the results of ultrasonographic examination at 18–20 weeks' gestation may be unacceptable. In addition, the skeletal findings in a compound heterozygote (for achondroplasia and hypochondroplasia) may not be evident that early in gestation because it is a milder phenotype than homozygous achondroplasia.

In vitro fertilization (IVF) and preimplantation genetic diagnosis could help this couple avoid the birth of a child who is a compound or double heterozygote by selecting embryos that have not inherited the wife's *FGFR3* gene mutation. Such embryos would have a 50% chance of having heterozygous hypochondroplasia like the husband, and a 50% chance of having normal stature. However, because of technical problems or unpredictable biological phenomenon, preimplantation genetic diagnosis is associated with a few percent error rate and confirmation of the results by chorionic villus sampling is recommended.

Whether to proceed with in vitro fertilization and preimplantation genetic diagnosis requires consideration about the associated risks and costs. There are preliminary data which suggest that manipulation of the sperm and egg by IVF may interfere with crucial genetic processes, resulting in a small increased risk of birth defects or rare genetic disorders. There continues to be ongoing investigation and surveillance of pregnancies conceived by these methods. A comprehensive review of the published experience thus far suggests that there is an increased risk ($\sim$1%) of abnormal outcomes associated with IVF with or without intracytoplasmic sperm injection compared to naturally conceived pregnancies. Some caution about these conclusions is warranted however, because available datasets are still relatively small and some studies have methodological limitations.

Special considerations in counseling individuals with skeletal dysplasias

Although individuals with achondroplasia or other similar skeletal dysplasias have more medical problems than individuals with average stature, normal intelligence is expected and most lead productive and satisfying lives. Terms such as "abnormal" and "disorder" when referring to the heterozygous state of achondroplasia (or other similar skeletal dysplasias) should be avoided. When discussing stature, some suggest using the term "average height" when referring to individuals of normal stature.

Further reading

1 Flynn M, Pauli, R (2003) Double heterozygosity in bone growth disorders: four new observations and review. *American Journal of Medical Genetics* **121A**: 193–208.

2 Francomano C (Updated 1/9/2006). Achondroplasia. In: *GeneReviews* at GeneTests: Medical Genetics Information Resource (database online). Copyright, University of Washington, Seattle. 1997–2009. Available at http://www.genetests.org. Accessed 9/2009.

3 Francomano C (Updated 12/12/2005). Hypochondroplasia. In: *GeneReviews* at GeneTests: Medical Genetics Information Resource (database online). Copyright, University of Washington, Seattle. 1997–2009. Available at http://www.genetests.org. Accessed 9/2009.

4 Gooding HC, Boehm K, Thompson RE *et al.* (2002) Issues surrounding prenatal genetic testing for achondroplasia. *Prenatal Diagnosis* **22**:933–940.

5 Hansen M, Bower C, Milne E *et al.* (2005) Assisted reproductive technologies and the risk of birth defects – a systematic review *Human Reproduction* **20**(2): 328–338.

6 Sommer A, Young-Wee T, Frye T (1987) Achondroplasia-hypochondroplasia complex. *American Journal of Medical Genetics* **26**:949–957.

Osteogenesis imperfecta

A couple is referred for genetic counseling because an ultrasonographic examination at 18 weeks' gestation reveals that the fetus has multiple fractures of the long bones, small beaded ribs, and diminished ossification of the calvarium. The husband reports that his wife from a previous marriage had a pregnancy which resulted in a stillbirth at 28 weeks' gestation. This fetus had a large head and severely shortened and abnormally shaped long bones. An autopsy was declined and there was no further investigation into the etiology.

Beaded ribs is the classic finding in osteogenesis imperfecta type II (OI type II). Other features of this perinatal lethal form of osteogenesis imperfecta include multiple fractures of the long bones resulting in severely deformed crumpled bones, platyspondyly, and hypomineralization of the skull. Death usually occurs within a few hours or days of life; there are rare long-term survivors who need intensive respiratory support. In utero fetal death also occurs.

OI type II is the most severe form of a group of disorders collectively known as osteogenesis imperfecta. Main features are varying degrees of bone fragility and in some forms, blue sclera, hearing loss, and abnormalities of dentition. The clinical spectrum of the disorder ranges from the severe perinatal lethal form (OI type II), to individuals with multiple severe deforming and disabling fractures, to individuals with a mild predisposition to fracture without significant health problems. The underlying biochemical abnormality in types I, II, III, and IV is a quantitative or qualitative defect of type I collagen which is the major protein component of bone and tendons.

Recurrence of OI type II among siblings is not uncommon and until the biochemical and molecular basis of the disorder was elucidated, the inheritance was incorrectly labeled as autosomal recessive. However, once the molecular defect of OI type II was understood, it became clear that autosomal dominant mutations in either the *COL1A1* or *COL1A2* genes, which alter the structure of either pro α1(I) or pro α2(I) chains of type I collagen, account for the vast majority of cases.

Therefore, gonadal or somatic mosaicism for a *COL1A1* or *COL1A2* gene mutation in one of the parents, rather than autosomal recessive inheritance, is the explanation for the recurrences that were observed among siblings. Empiric data show that once a couple has had a child with OI type II, the risk of recurrence in a subsequent pregnancy is about 7%. Some couples face a higher risk if one of the parents has somatic or gonadal mosaicism for a *COL1A1* or *COL1A2* gene mutation, while other couples have a much lower risk if the mutation causing disease in their affected child arose as a de novo event in a single sperm or ovum. Differentiating between these possibilities after a couple has had one affected child is usually not possible.

The ultrasonographic findings in the husband's first wife's pregnancy are strongly suspicious for OI type II and the findings in the current pregnancy are almost diagnostic. There are other disorders which in utero have some features of OI type II that should be excluded. These include achondrogenesis, hypophosphatasia, and thanatophoric dysplasia. A definitive diagnosis could be made if a mutation were identified in one of the fetal *COL1A1* or *COL1A2* genes. This would also enable preimplantation genetic diagnosis or early prenatal diagnosis in a future pregnancy. In the rare families where a molecular defect is not identified, collagen synthesis studies could be performed on cultured fibroblasts as almost all infants with OI type II make an abnormal species of type I collagen that can be identified by gel electrophoresis, or produce a deficient amount of type I collagen.

Analysis of DNA obtained from cultured fetal skin fibroblasts after pregnancy termination documents a point mutation in one COL1A2 gene, confirming the diagnosis of OI type II in the fetus.

The husband has fathered two babies with different partners who had or are strongly suspected of having OI type II. He could have gonadal or somatic mosaicism for a *COL1A2* gene mutation.

The husband reports that he is significantly shorter than his siblings. Physical examination reveals only mild dentinogenesis imperfecta. He is athletic and has never had a fracture.

The husband's physical findings suggest that he has somatic mosaicism for a *COL1A2* gene mutation. Analysis of DNA obtained from his skin fibroblasts confirmed that he is mosaic. Although his mutation has not caused any clinical sequela other than dentinogenesis imperfecta and possible short stature, it has had significant reproductive consequences.

Accurately predicting the chance of another recurrence of OI type II in a future pregnancy is difficult to make. If a high fraction of the husband's sperm has the *COL1A2* gene mutation, the risk of recurrence could approach 50%. Quantitative analysis of DNA from sperm might theoretically provide some useful information but empiric evidence for this approach is not available.

In a future pregnancy, preimplantation or prenatal genetic diagnosis could be used. For prenatal diagnosis, either molecular analysis or sonographic imaging would establish a diagnosis. Because the disease-causing mutation has been identified, definitive prenatal diagnosis by chorionic villus sampling beginning at 10 to 11 weeks' gestation can be done. Alternatively, if the couple wishes to avoid the risks associated with an invasive diagnostic procedure, ultrasonographic examination performed by an experienced sonographer would be satisfactory in most instances because the skeletal abnormalities of OI type II are usually apparent by 13–14 weeks' gestation. Given that results of molecular analysis of DNA obtained from chorionic villi are usually available in 1–2 weeks, relying on ultrasonographic information alone would not add significantly to the waiting time to obtain diagnostic information.

In a family in which a *COL1A1* or *COL1A2* gene mutation has not been identified but abnormal collagen synthesis has been documented, prenatal diagnosis could be accomplished by collagen synthesis studies of cultured chorionic villus cells.

Further reading

1 Byers PH, Tsipouras P, Bonadio JF *et al.* (1988) Perinatal lethal osteogenesis imperfecta (OI type II): a biochemically heterogeneous disorder usually due to new mutations in the genes for type I collagen. *American Journal of Human Genetics* **42**(2): 237–248.

2 Cohn DH, Starman BJ, Blumberg B *et al.* (1991) Recurrence of lethal osteogenesis imperfecta due to parental mosaicism for a dominant mutation in human type I collagen gene. *American Journal of Human Genetics* **46**:591–601.

3 DiMaio MS, Barth R, Koprivnikar KE *et al.* (1993) First trimester prenatal diagnosis of osteogenesis imperfecta type II by DNA analysis and sonography. *Prenatal Diagnosis* **13**:589–596.

4 Hsieh CT, Yeh GP, Wu HH *et al.* (2008) Fetus with osteogenesis imperfecta presenting as increased nuchal translucency thickness in the first trimester. *Journal of Clinical Ultrasound* **36**:119–122.

5 Steiner RD, Pepin MG, Byers PH (Updated 1/28/2005). Osteogenesis Imperfecta. In: *GeneReviews* at Gene Tests: Medical Genetics Information Resource (database online). Copyright, University of Washington, Seattle. 1997–2009. Available at http://www.genetests.org.

6 Zlotogora J (1998) Germ line mosaicism. *Human Genetics* **102**(4):381–386.

Short rib polydactyly syndrome

A 28-year-old woman is referred for genetic counseling. Her family history is remarkable for her daughter who died in the neonatal period of abnormalities consistent with short rib polydactyly syndrome. The woman and her husband are first cousins. She has had four first trimester miscarriages. The peripheral blood karyotype for the daughter with short rib polydactyly was 46,XX, t(7;15) (q22;p11.2) consistent with an apparently balanced translocation between the long arm of chromosome 7 and the short arm of chromosome 15. Array comparative genomic hybridization did not detect any variants, deletions, or insertions of genetic material. The woman has the same 7;15 chromosomal translocation. Her husband has a normal peripheral blood karyotype. The woman's family history includes a brother who has mental retardation of unknown cause.

In addition to ova that contain a normal haploid or balanced chromosomal complement, this woman will produce ova with various combinations of unbalanced haploid complements involving partial monosomies and trisomies for chromosomes 7 and 15. The effects on the embryo of an unbalanced translocation depend on the various combinations of extra or missing genetic material. Conceptuses with a large amount of extra (partial trisomy) or missing (partial monosomy) genetic material

would likely die early in embryogenesis, often before a pregnancy is recognized. Monosomies or trisomies involving small amounts of genetic material are often compatible with viability and survival after birth and often are associated with mental retardation of variable severity and abnormalities of major organ systems.

The translocation involves chromosomes 7 and 15, chromosomes which contain imprinted genes. There is a small increased risk of uniparental disomy for chromosomes 7 and/or 15 which, if present, would be associated with abnormalities of varying severity. This risk is estimated at less than 1%.

In addition, the couple has had a child with short rib polydactyly syndrome (SRPS) which is a genetically heterogeneous group of lethal autosomal recessive disorders whose major features include markedly shortened ribs leading to thoracic hypoplasia, short limbs, polydactyly, and abnormalities of major organs. The molecular defect of only one form of SRPS has been identified. For the majority of families who have had a child with SRPS the disease-causing mutation(s) are unknown at present. This couple is consanguineous which suggests that both members of the couple carry the same mutation in a SRPS gene.

An alternative hypothesis is that the chromosomal translocation played a role in causing SRPS in the couple's child. Although the translocation appeared unassociated with a deletion or duplication of genetic material in the child, one of the breakpoints may disrupt a SRPS-related gene. If her husband had an *SRPS* mutation at the locus involved in his wife's translocation, and he transmitted that gene to the affected child, the child would have had two abnormal *SRPS* genes and manifest disease. Whether there is an association in this family between the translocation and SRPS cannot be answered at present and must await more insights into the molecular basis of the SRPS group of disorders. Regardless of whether the two findings are related, the risk of recurrence of short rib polydactyly in the current pregnancy is 25%.

The couple's consanguinity adds additional risks. The offspring of first cousin marriages face a risk of birth defects and mental retardation which is 5–6% or about double that faced by the offspring of unrelated parents. This is in addition to the 25% risk of recurrence of a child with SRPS. Many of these disorders would not be evident on ultrasonographic examination. Because the woman's brother has mental retardation, there is also an increased risk of recurrence of his problems in the current pregnancy due to the consanguineous mating or the translocation.

The woman has also had four first-trimester miscarriages. These early pregnancy losses might be the consequence of a fetus with an unbalanced 7;15 translocation. They may also reflect the increased risk of pregnancy wastage among consanguineous couples due to homozygosity for lethal genetic conditions.

In a future pregnancy, further testing can include chorionic villus sampling to determine the chromosomal status of the fetus and whether there is biparental inheritance for chromosomes 7 and 15. Beginning at 13–14 weeks' gestation, ultrasonographic examinations should be performed every few weeks to look for the skeletal findings associated with SRPS. Manifestation of some forms of SRPS may be identifiable by ultrasonographic examination as early as 13 weeks' gestation. By 20 weeks' gestation, the majority of affected fetuses would have sonographic findings.

There are no satisfactory ways to address the other risks associated with the couple's consanguinity. Ultrasonographic imaging will identify gross structural defects but many single gene and multifactorial disorders do not have manifestations until after birth. With respect to the woman's brother's mental retardation, no specific testing can be offered unless the underlying cause of his problems has been identified. Ideally, a complete genetics evaluation of the brother should be performed. At the very least,

photographs and information about his clinical presentation should be obtained. Fragile X syndrome carrier testing should be offered to the woman because fragile X syndrome is a common inherited cause of mental retardation.

If the woman experiences another spontaneous pregnancy loss, efforts should be made to karyotype the products of conception.

Further reading

1 Elçioglu NH, Hall CM (2002) Diagnostic dilemmas in the short rib-polydactyly syndrome group. *American Journal of Medical Genetics* **111**:392–400.

2 Franceschini P, Guala A, Vardeu MP *et al.* (1995) Short rib-dysplasia group (with/without polydactyly): report of a patient suggesting the existence of a continuous spectrum. *American Journal of Medical Genetics* **59**: 359–364.

3 Merrill AE, Merriman B, Farrington-Rock C *et al.* (2009) Ciliary abnormalities due to defects in the retrograde transport protein DYNC2H1 in short-rib polydactyly syndrome. *American Journal of Human Genetics* **84**:542–549.

3   Non-Mendelian Inheritance

Prenatal Diagnosis: Cases & Clinical Challenges, 1st edition.   By Miriam S. DiMaio, Joyce E. Fox, Maurice J. Mahoney
Published 2010 by Blackwell Publishing Ltd.

Introduction to non-Mendelian inheritance

Non-Mendelian disorders have patterns of inheritance which do not conform to Mendel's Law of Segregation where each ovum or sperm receives only one copy of a pair of genes. Important examples include mitochondrial inheritance, genetic imprinting, and multifactorial inheritance.

Mitochondrial disorders can be caused by abnormalities in either nuclear genes or in mitochondrial DNA. Mitochondrial disorders caused by abnormalities of nuclear genes are inherited in a Mendelian fashion. Mutations in mitochondrial DNA (mtDNA) cause disorders which have mitochondrial inheritance. An important feature of disorders with mitochondrial inheritance is heteroplasmy, i.e., varying amounts of mutant and normal mtDNA in each cell. Mitochondrial DNA is almost exclusively maternally transmitted; hence, mitochondrial disorders do not follow Mendel's Law of Segregation as all children of an affected mother will inherit abnormal mtDNA. The manifestations of disorders with mitochondrial inheritance may vary widely among affected offspring because different amounts of normal and mutant mtDNA are present in each ovum.

Genetic imprinting is responsible for another class of non-Mendelian disorders. Several imprinted genes are normally expressed or silenced depending on whether they have been paternally or maternally transmitted. Chemical modifications to the gene structure but not the gene sequence lead to this phenomenon. Risk of recurrence of an imprinted disorder depends on the specific genetic mechanism leading to aberrant gene imprinting and the parent of origin.

Disorders with multifactorial inheritance are caused by the effects and complex interactions of multiple susceptibility genes, each usually with a relatively small effect, and environmental and epigenetic factors. Multifactorial conditions constitute a significant fraction of common birth defects such as congenital heart disease, neural tube defects, facial clefting, and common medical problems such as diabetes, autoimmune disease, cancer, and most cases of autistic spectrum disorder. This class of non-Mendelian disorders is the most etiologically complex and poorly understood. While multiple members of the same family are sometimes affected, multifactorial disorders are not associated with Mendelian patterns of inheritance.

Mitochondrial inheritance

Features of mitochondrial inheritance

1 Mitochondrial DNA (mtDNA) is almost exclusively maternal in origin; there is a negligible contribution from sperm.
2 There is exclusive maternal transmission.
3 Only maternal offspring are affected.
4 Males and females are equally likely to be affected.
5 No transmission occurs to descendants of affected males.
6 Phenotypic predictions are complicated by heteroplasmy (mixture of normal and abnormal mtDNA).

Mitochondrial disorders

A couple is referred for genetic counseling because their 14-month-old daughter has just been diagnosed with Leigh syndrome. Over the past several months, she had regression of motor skills with onset of abnormal movements, progressive hypotonia, irritability, and loss of appetite with vomiting. Seizures began at 10 months of age and symptoms seemed to worsen in association with viral illnesses. She has elevated lactate concentrations in blood and cerebrospinal fluid. Brain imaging showed multiple spongiform lesions in specific areas of the brain, which are findings characteristic of Leigh syndrome. The wife, age 33 years, is now 10 weeks pregnant.

Leigh syndrome, one of a number of mitochondrial disorders associated with defective energy metabolism, is a neurodegenerative disorder which results from a deficiency of any of the mitochondrial respiratory chain complexes. Mutations in a number of different genes with different inheritance patterns can lead to the Leigh syndrome phenotype.

About 70% of cases of Leigh syndrome are associated with mutations in nuclear DNA (nDNA) and have autosomal or X-linked inheritance patterns (i.e., they are inherited as autosomal recessive, autosomal dominant, or X-linked conditions). The remaining 30% of cases are attributed to mutations in mitochondrial DNA (mtDNA) and have an inheritance pattern which is characteristic of mitochondrial inheritance.

Mitochondrial inheritance differs from Mendelian inheritance because functioning mitochondria and the mtDNA within them are inherited exclusively from one's mother. If a woman has a mitochondrial disorder due to a mtDNA mutation, each of her children, regardless of sex, has close to a 100% chance of inheriting the disorder if the mutant mtDNA are present in her ova. However, the severity of disease expression in her children may be highly variable due to differing amounts of mutant mtDNA load. Normal mitochondrial functioning and a normal phenotype may be present if the mutant mtDNA load is below a certain threshold. Males with mitochondrial disorders due to mutant mtDNA do not transmit the disorder to their children. Evidence for transmission of disease from males to their offspring essentially excludes mitochondrial inheritance from consideration.

A mitochondrial disorder caused by a mtDNA mutation may arise de novo in the mitochondria of an affected child. Almost always, however, mitochondrial disorders due to mtDNA mutations are transmitted from the mother who also has the mtDNA mutation. She will usually be asymptomatic or less severely affected.

There is a wide continuum of disease severity within and among families affected by mitochondrial disorders due to mtDNA mutations. This is largely accounted for by heteroplasmy, the situation in which there is more than one type of mtDNA present within each cell. Hundreds of copies of mitochondria and mitochondrial DNA are present in each human cell.

The burden of mutant mtDNA varies between cells and among different tissues. A high burden of mutant mtDNA will usually result in early onset and severe disease. A low burden of mutant mtDNA may be compatible with a normal phenotype, with milder symptoms, or with onset of symptoms later in life. In addition to heteroplasmy, the nature of the mutation itself will also influence the severity of disease expression of mitochondrial disorders.

Once the disorder is suspected from the clinical presentation, further diagnostic testing may include brain imaging, metabolic studies of blood and cerebrospinal fluid, histopathology of muscle biopsy, and respiratory chain enzyme studies of tissue biopsies.

Establishing the molecular basis of a mitochondrial disorder will provide information about recurrence risk in future children, allow for prenatal diagnosis in future pregnancies, and permit the identification of at-risk relatives. However, molecular testing is complicated by the extensive genetic heterogeneity of Leigh syndrome; at least six autosomal genes and 11 mitochondrial genes are associated with the syndrome. Furthermore, for some mtDNA mutations that cause Leigh syndrome, the percentage of abnormal mtDNA may vary between different tissues and may decrease in white blood cells with increasing age. Analysis of mtDNA obtained from skeletal muscle or urine sediment is associated with the highest sensitivity in the detection of mtDNA mutations for Leigh syndrome. For analysis of nDNA mutations when a nuclear mitochondrial disorder is suspected, DNA obtained from leukocytes is satisfactory.

Obtaining information about the family may provide clues as to the mode of inheritance and can help direct the strategy for molecular testing. For disorders due to mtDNA mutations, affected relatives on the maternal side may have symptoms that have not been recognized as part of the disease spectrum. In the absence of a family history that suggests a mitochondrial disorder, an autosomal recessive disorder or a de novo autosomal dominant disorder would be possibilities.

A family history is collected. Neither parent reports relatives with neurodegenerative disorders. The father of the child with Leigh syndrome is in good health. The mother's health history is remarkable only for migraine headaches. Her brother developed night blindness in his late teens and is thought to have retinitis pigmentosa. He has four children who are healthy. The maternal grandmother died at age 62 years shortly after being diagnosed with a cardiac arrhythmia.

The mother's health and family history suggest that a mtDNA mutation could be the underlying cause for her daughter's Leigh syndrome. Migraine headaches, night blindness, diabetes, cardiac conduction defects leading to sudden unexpected death, and muscle weakness are included in the spectrum of clinical problems that can be seen in the mothers and other maternal relatives of a child with Leigh syndrome.

Mutations in one of the mtDNA genes causing Leigh syndrome can also lead to another disorder known as NARP (**n**eurogenic muscle weakness, **a**taxia, and **r**etinitis **p**igmentosa). Other features of NARP which may be present include short stature, sensorineural hearing loss, progressive external ophthalmoplegia, and cardiac conduction defects. The symptoms of NARP often begin in early childhood, may remain stable for many years, may be exacerbated by viral illnesses, or may not be appreciated until adulthood. In some families, affected individuals may have classic Leigh syndrome, NARP, or any combination of the features of these disorders.

Analysis of mtDNA obtained from the affected daughter's skeletal muscle revealed a mtDNA mutation associated with both Leigh syndrome and NARP. This mutation was subsequently documented in the mother and her brother. The couple wants prenatal diagnosis of Leigh syndrome in the current pregnancy.

Each of the couple's children will inherit both mutant and wildtype mtDNA from the mother that will be present in varying proportions. A number of different options are available to decrease transmission of mtDNA mutations (see Table 3.1). The ratios of wildtype and mutant DNA

Table 3.1 Strengths and weaknesses of reproductive options for preventing transmission of mtDNA mutations

	CVS or aminocyte analysis	Preimplantation genetic diagnosis	Nuclear or cytoplasmic transfer	Donor oocyte IVF
Cost and simplicity of procedure	***	*	?	**
Likelihood of achieving a pregnancy	***	*	?	**
Ability of parents to access the procedure	***	**	?	*
Avoidance of pregnancy termination	*	***	**	***
Ease of data interpretation	*	**	*	***
Situations where procedure may be suitable	Women with low recurrence risk[a]	Women with low to moderate loads	Not yet recommended but may be suited to women with high mutant loads	Women with moderate to high mutant loads

CVS, chorionic villus sampling; IFV, in vitro fertilization.
*weaknesses.
**intermediate.
***strengths.
[a]Examples include women with (1) a very low mutant load (<10%) of certain mutations in blood or other tissues, (2) a very low mutant load (<10%) of certain mtDNA point mutations in skeletal muscle, (3) a single mtDNA deletion and no detectable duplicated mtDNA in skeletal muscle, and (4) the majority of oocytes lacking mutant mtDNA, as shown by preimplantation genetic diagnosis or oocyte sampling.
Reproduced from Thorburn DR, Dahl HH (2001) Amercian Journal of Medical Genetics (Seminars in Medical Genetics) **106**:102–114 with permission from John Wiley and Sons, Inc.

present in uncultured chorionic villi or amniocytes reflect the mutant load present in most tissues at birth. Attempts have been made to predict the severity of disease in a fetus based on the proportions of mutant and wildtype mtDNA. These predictions should be made cautiously but appear, at least for Leigh syndrome, to provide reasonable guidance if there are very high or very low proportions of mtDNA in the fetal sample. Prior to initiating prenatal diagnosis, couples should be aware that predictions about the phenotypic outcome would not be possible when the proportions of mutant and wildtype mtDNA are roughly equivalent. Analysis of mtDNA for prenatal diagnosis should be performed on uncultured chorionic villi or amniocytes due to the possibility that the proportions of wildtype and mutant mtDNA will change during cell culture.

In vitro fertilization with preimplantation genetic diagnosis would also be possible for future pregnancies. Only embryos which have a very low or preferably zero mutant load should be used for implantation. In vitro fertilization using an ovum from a donor who is not a maternal relative of the wife would be another alternative to avoid the risk of having a child affected by Leigh syndrome. Research has also showed the feasibility of using the nucleus of a woman's ovum and cytoplasm with mitochondria from another woman's ovum for the maternal contribution to a conceptus.

Further reading

1 Bredenoord AL, Pennings G, Smeets HJ *et al.* (2008) Dealing with uncertainties: ethics of prenatal diagnosis and preimplantation genetic diagnosis to prevent mitochondrial disorders. *Human Reproduction Update* **14**:83–94.

2 Thorburn DR, Dahl, HH. (2001) Mitochondrial disorders: genetics, counseling, prenatal diagnosis and reproductive options. *American Journal of Medical Genetics (Seminars in Medical Genetics)* **106**:102–114.

Imprinting disorders

The parents of a 4-year-old girl who may have Angelman syndrome are seen for genetic counseling. The daughter has the characteristic findings of the disorder which include developmental delay that became apparent in the first year of life, severe mental retardation, absent speech, a distinctive facial appearance, hand flapping, and an unusually happy demeanor. She also has microcephaly and seizures that are commonly seen in Angelman syndrome. The mother is pregnant and wants to know the risk of recurrence of her daughter's problems and whether prenatal diagnosis is available. The couple has two other children who are developmentally normal. The daughter's diagnosis has not been confirmed by molecular testing. The mother is 8 weeks pregnant.

Angelman syndrome is a disorder resulting from abnormal genetic imprinting of the *UBE3A* gene on chromosome 15q11.2-q13. Imprinting occurs when the parental origin of a gene determines whether or not it is expressed. Only a small minority of human genes are subject to imprinting effects. Imprinting results from epigenetic phenomena in which gene expression is controlled by DNA methylation and other chemical processes that alter the DNA but not the gene sequence. In general, genes that are methylated are silenced and demethylation results in activation of gene expression. In each generation, reprogramming (methylation or demethylation) of imprinted genes occurs in ova and sperm. The sex of the transmitting parent determines whether or not an imprinted gene will be expressed or silenced in the next generation, regardless of whether that gene was expressed in that parent.

In normal individuals, only the maternally inherited *UBE3A* gene is expressed while the paternally inherited allele is silenced. Angelman syndrome arises due to loss of expression of the maternally inherited *UBE3A* allele, which can be a consequence of different genetic processes that include the following.

1 A chromosomal deletion at chromosome 15q11.2-q13 on the maternally inherited allele accounts for about 70% of cases. Most are de novo. Almost all are microdeletions that cannot be detected by routine metaphase karyotyping but can be found by fluorescence in situ hybridization (FISH) or array comparative genomic hybridization (array CGH). In rare cases, microdeletions are found in association with either de novo or inherited chromosomal rearrangements involving the 15q11.2-q13 locus.

2 Seven percent of cases are due to paternal uniparental disomy for chromosome 15, where both copies of chromosome 15 are from the father and there is absence of the maternally inherited chromosome 15. Uniparental disomy can be detected by analysis of DNA polymorphisms on chromosome 15 in the affected child and parents and by other molecular techniques.

3 Three percent of cases are due to a 6–200 kb microdeletion in the imprinting center of the *UBE3A* gene on the maternally inherited chromosome which results in silencing of the gene. This explanation is inferred if aberrant gene methylation is present and a chromosomal deletion and uniparental disomy have been excluded.

4 Another 11% of cases have a point mutation in or deletion of the entire *UBE3A* gene which can be detected by gene sequencing or other molecular methods used to detect chromosomal deletions.

5 At this time, an underlying genetic abnormality is not found in about 11% of individuals with the clinical diagnosis of Angelman syndrome. This may be due to an incorrect clinical diagnosis, or other unidentified genetic mechanisms resulting in aberrant *UBE3A* gene function or expression.

Chromosomal microdeletions, uniparental disomy, and *UBE3A* gene imprinting center defects are all associated with abnormal DNA methylation. However, abnormal DNA methylation does not establish the underlying molecular basis of the disorder, information which is important for providing information about the risk of recurrence and accurate prenatal diagnosis. If abnormal DNA methylation is present, array CGH or FISH should be performed to look for a chromosomal deletion. If a chromosome deletion is found, a metaphase karyotype should be obtained to look for a chromosome rearrangement. If FISH or array CGH is normal, uniparental disomy studies should be performed. If uniparental disomy is not found, further molecular studies could be performed to identify a small microdeletion or other change in the imprinting center of the *UBE3A* gene.

If DNA methylation studies are normal, *UBE3A* gene sequence analysis is indicated.

Risk of recurrence of Angelman syndrome varies widely depending on the underlying molecular pathogenesis. As shown in Table 3.2, risk of recurrence is small unless a parent carries a chromosomal rearrangement involving chromosome 15, or if the mother herself carries a *UBE3A* gene mutation or imprinting center defect. (For these latter possibilities, the mother herself could be unaffected by Angelman syndrome because the *UBE3A* gene mutation could either have been transmitted from her father or have arisen de novo on her paternally inherited chromosome 15.) For de novo mutations in the child, the risk of

Table 3.2 Genetic mechanisms in Angelman syndrome (AS) and Prader–Willi syndrome (PWS) and risk of recurrence in the siblings of an affected child

Genetic mechanism	Percentage of families	Recurrence risk
Deletion of 15q11-q13	70 (both AS and PW)	<1%
UPD of chromosome 15	~25 (PWS) 3–7 (AS)	<1%
Mutation in UBE3A	~10 (AS)	50% if present in mother
No identifiable molecular abnormality	~10 (AS)	Unknown
Imprinting center defect without mutation in the imprinting center	1–3 (both)	<1%
Imprinting center defect with mutation in the imprinting center	<1 (both)	50% if present in father (PWS) or mother (AS)
De novo unbalanced rearrangement of 15q11-q13	<1 (both)	<1%
Inherited unbalanced rearrangement of 15q11-q13	<1 (both)	≤50%
UPD due to parental rearrangement involving chromosome 15	<1 (both)	Depends on translocation; if parent has 15;15 Robertsonian translocation, risk would approach 100%; for most others, risk is ≤0.75%

UPD, uniparental disomy.
Data from Williams CA, Dagli AI, Driscoll DJ (Updated 9/5/2008). Angelman syndrome. In: Gene Reviews at GeneTests: Medical Genetics Information Resource (database online). Copyright, University of Washington, Seattle. 1997–2009. Available at http://www.genetests.org. Accessed September 2009; Cassidy SB, Schwartz S (Updated 3/24/2008). Prader-Willi syndrome. In: Gene Reviews at GeneTests: Medical Genetics Information Resource (database online). Copyright, University of Washington, Seattle. 1997–2009. Available at http://www. genetests.org. Accessed September 2009. Table adapted from Kokkonen H. (2003) Genetic changes of chromosome region 15q11–q13 in Prader-Willi and Angelman syndromes in Finland http://herkules.oulu.fi/isbn9514270274/html/index.html

recurrence is very small, but not zero because of the possibility of gonadal mosaicism.

Array CGH reveals a microdeletion at the chromosome 15q12 locus, confirming the clinical diagnosis of Angelman syndrome. Routine cytogenetic analysis of the daughter reveals an apparently balanced translocation between chromosomes 4p16 and 15q12.

The translocation could have arisen as a de novo event or have been inherited from one of the parents who are both phenotypically normal.

The father has a normal karyotype. The mother has a balanced translocation between chromosomes 4p16 and 15q12. Array CGH does not show any evidence for a deletion or duplication of genetic material.

The daughter inherited her mother's chromosomal translocation which, in contrast to the mother, also has a small interstitial deletion on chromosome 15 resulting in absence of a functional maternally derived *UBE3A* gene. The identification of the chromosomal translocation in the mother has implications both for recurrence of conceptuses who have unbalanced translocations involving partial trisomies and monosomies for chromosomes 4 and 15 and Angelman syndrome due to an interstitial deletion at the 15q12 locus.

This family is an example of the rare circumstance in which the same apparently balanced translocation is associated with a normal phenotype in one relative and an abnormal phenotype in another due to a de novo structural alteration, in this case an interstitial deletion at one of the translocation breakpoints. In the current pregnancy, the risk of recurrence of another child who has inherited the mother's apparently balanced translocation *and* also has a microdeletion at the chromosome 15q12 locus is very small. This risk is far outweighed by the significant chance of a child with an unbalanced chromosomal translocation.

For individuals who carry either a reciprocal or Robertsonian translocation involving chromosome 15, there is also a small additional risk of uniparental disomy for chromosome 15 resulting from malsegregation of the chromosomes involved in the translocation during meiosis. This could lead to some gametes with two copies of chromosome 15 and some gametes with no copy of chromosome 15. Uniparental disomy for chromosome 15 can arise via two mechanisms. The more likely situation would be trisomy rescue in which an embryo with trisomy 15 is "rescued" by loss of a chromosome 15 after fertilization, resulting in a karyotypically normal fetus who now has two copies of either the maternally or paternally derived chromosome 15. Another, less likely, situation would be a zygote conceived with one gamete with disomy for chromosome 15 and another which was nullisomic for chromosome 15. Both of these situations could result in absence of either the maternally or paternally inherited chromosome 15, leading to Angelman syndrome or Prader–Willi syndrome, respectively. The risk of uniparental disomy in the setting of a parent with a balanced translocation is estimated at 0.7%.

If other maternal relatives carry the translocation, they would face similar risks.

> *The woman's brother, who is healthy and developmentally normal, is referred for consultation because he also carries the chromosome translocation between chromosomes 4p16 and 15q12. Array CGH does not detect a duplication or deletion of genetic material.*

This man is at significant risk for conceiving children who have unbalanced chromosomal complements involving various combinations of partial monosomies and partial trisomies for chromosomes 4 and 15. In addition, there would be a very small additional risk of a child with a de novo submicroscopic interstitial deletion at the site of one of the translocation breakpoints as discovered in his niece. Such a deletion on chromosome 15q12 would not result in Angelman syndrome because it would be of paternal origin and the affected child would still have a functional maternally inherited *UBE3A* gene. However, the 15q11.2q13 locus also contains the Prader–Willi critical region (PWCR) which contains genes which are subject to imprinting effects. Genetic abnormalities in the paternally derived PWCR will result in Prader–Willi syndrome. The main features of Prader–Willi syndrome include neonatal and infantile hypotonia and feeding problems, mild to moderate mental retardation, hyperphagia during childhood leading to obesity, short stature, small hands and feet, hypogonadism, and distinctive facial features.

Almost all individuals with Prader–Willi syndrome have an imprinting defect in the PWCR which is caused by one of several mechanisms leading to loss of expression of genes in the paternally derived PWCR. About 75% of cases have chromosomal microdeletions on the paternally derived allele (associated with abnormal DNA methylation and also diagnosable by FISH or array CGH). Maternal disomy for chromosome 15 (associated with abnormal DNA methylation and diagnosable by

molecular analysis) is present in about 25% of cases. Less than 1% of cases are due to an imprinting center defect in the paternally derived chromosome. Imprinting center defects can be caused by microdeletions in the paternal PWCR imprinting center, which are associated with abnormal DNA methylation and can be detected by gene sequencing, or, more commonly, they can be due to abnormalities of gene methylation of the paternal allele which are not associated with a gene sequence change. While abnormal methylation confirms the clinical diagnosis of Prader–Willi syndrome, establishing the underlying molecular basis for the disorder is important for recurrence risk counseling and accurate prenatal diagnosis.

As shown in Table 3.2, inherited chromosomal rearrangements are a rare cause of Angelman syndrome and Prader–Willi syndrome and the presence of both disorders in the same family is an extremely unusual situation.

> *The mother who carries the balanced reciprocal translocation between chromosomes 4p16 and 15q12 elects to undergo chorionic villus sampling based on the increased risk of conceptuses with unbalanced chromosomal complements and the chance of recurrence of the microdeletion at the chromosome 15q12 locus. The karyotype of cultured chorionic villus cells reveals that the fetus inherited the mother's apparently balanced translocation between chromosomes 4p16 and 15q12.*

As noted above, most microdeletions causing Angelman syndrome, including the one found in the woman's affected daughter, cannot be detected by routine metaphase karyotyping. Two approaches, FISH or array CGH, can be used to investigate the possibility of a submicroscopic microdeletion at the Angelman syndrome locus on chromosome 15q12. FISH uses probes specific for this locus and would address the presence of absence of a deletion (or duplication) at the Angelman syndrome locus only. However, this woman's reciprocal translocation also involves a breakpoint on chromosome 4p16. Inherited balanced rearrangements are rarely associated with submicroscopic de novo duplications or deletions resulting in an abnormal phenotype, although this did occur at the chromosome 15q12 locus for the daughter. Array CGH of DNA obtained from cultured or uncultured chorionic villi would also address this risk of a duplication or deletion of genetic material at the chromosome 4p16 locus, as well as the 15q12 locus. Because the early embryo and placenta are hypomethylated, it is not yet certain whether DNA methylation studies would be reliable in the first trimester.

Within the limits of the technology, array CGH did not detect a deletion or duplication at the breakpoints of the translocation on chromosomes 4 and 15 or elsewhere in the fetal genome.

Because the maternal translocation involving chromosome 15 has a small chance of resulting in maternal uniparental disomy for chromosome 15, which causes Prader–Willi syndrome, molecular studies are indicated to determine whether both parents have contributed a chromosome 15.

In future pregnancies, preimplantation genetic diagnosis using probes for the translocation and the typical Angelman syndrome deletion could be used. Whether uniparental disomy for chromosome 15 could be addressed at the same time would depend on available technology and experience in the laboratory. Because the early embryo is hypomethylated, preimplantation genetic diagnosis by methylation studies is not recommended.

Similar approaches could be used for the woman's brother and his wife for a future pregnancy to address the risks of a fetus with an unbalanced chromosomal translocation, the possibility of a microdeletion at chromosome 15q12 leading to Prader–Willi syndrome, and paternal uniparental disomy leading to Angelman syndrome.

Further reading

1 Cassidy SB, Schwartz S (Updated 3/24/2008) Prader-Willi syndrome. In: *GeneReviews* at GeneTests: Medical Genetics Information Resource (database online). Copyright, University of Washington, Seattle. 1997–2009. Available at http://www.genetests.org. Accessed September 2009.

2 Gurrieri F, Accadia M (2009) Genetic imprinting: the paradigm of Prader-Willi and Angelman syndromes. *Endocrine Development* **14**:20–28.

3 Horsthemke B, Maat-Kievit A, Sleegers E *et al.* (1996) Familial translocations involving 15q11-q13 can give rise to interstitial deletions causing Prader-Willi or Angelman syndrome. *Journal of Medical Genetics* **33**:848–851.

4 Knoll JH, Wagstaff J, Lalande M (1993) Cytogenetic and molecular studies in the Prader-Willi and Angelman syndromes: an overview. *American Journal of Medical Genetics* **46**(1):2–6.

5 Smeets, DFCM, Hamel BCJ, Nelen, MR *et al.* (1992) Prader-Willi syndrome and Angelman syndrome in cousins from a family with translocation between chromosomes 6 and 15. *New England Journal of Medicine* **326**(12):807–811.

6 Stalker HJ, Williams CA (1998) Genetic counseling in Angelman syndrome: the challenges of multiple causes. *American Journal of Medical Genetics* **77**: 54–59.

7 Williams CA, Dagli AI, Driscoll DJ (Updated 9/5/2008) Angelman syndrome. In: *GeneReviews* at GeneTests: Medical Genetics Information Resource (database online). Copyright, University of Washington, Seattle. 1997–2009. Available at http://www.genetests.org. Accessed September 2009.

Multifactorial inheritance

Features of multifactorial inheritance

1 The disorder is due to the interactions of one or more genes and environmental factors.

2 The risk of recurrence is highest among first-degree relatives of an affected individual and decreases markedly for relatives with greater than a second-degree relationship.

3 In the absence of empiric data, the risk of recurrence in a first-degree relative can be approximated by the square root of the incidence.

4 Risk of recurrence is higher when the affected individual is of the sex that is less frequently affected.

5 Risk of recurrence is increased if more than one family member is affected.

6 Risk of recurrence or severity of the disorder may be increased, or time of onset may be earlier, if the affected family member has severe expression of the disorder.

7 Disease incidence and recurrence risks may vary by ethnicity or geographic area.

Multifactorial disorders

A couple is referred for genetic counseling because the wife had repair of a unilateral cleft lip and palate. The husband's father has spina bifida with normal intelligence and the husband's maternal uncle had a congenital heart defect. The couple is not consanguineous and no other relatives have facial clefting, neural tube defects, or congenital heart disease. Each have three siblings who do not have congenital malformations.

Spina bifida, facial clefting, and congenital heart disease are structural malformations which usually have multifactorial inheritance. Multifactorial disorders arise due to the interactions of one or more genes and environmental factors. (Polygenic disorders are ones which result from the effects of multiple genes but where the influence of environmental factors is discounted.)

For multifactorial disorders, the major factor influencing risk of recurrence is the degree of relationship. First-degree relatives of an affected individual, whether parent or a sibling, will have the highest recurrence risk which, in the absence of empiric data, can be approximated by the square root of the incidence of the disorder. The risk of recurrence is usually slightly higher than the general population risk for second-degree relatives (the grandchild or niece or nephew of an affected individual). The risk of recurrence for third-degree relatives usually approaches that of the general population.

Another factor influencing recurrence risk is the severity of the abnormality in the affected individual. More severe manifestations may be associated with a higher recurrence risk, reflecting a higher degree of genetic loading or genetic liability (the presence of a greater number of susceptibility genes, or genes that have a lower threshold for being expressed), or the influence of unique environmental risk factor(s). For these reasons also, consanguinity between parents increases the risk of occurrence and recurrence of a multifactorial disorder.

Some multifactorial disorders occur more frequently in one sex than the other. The risk of recurrence will be higher if the affected sibling or parent is of the less commonly affected sex. This also reflects the presence of a higher degree of genetic loading that has resulted in disease expression in the sex which usually has lower susceptibility.

If more than one sibling is affected by a multifactorial disorder, this further increases the risk of recurrence in subsequent children. An affected first-degree relative usually confers a higher risk of recurrence than the presence of multiple affected relatives who are more distantly related.

Counseling about recurrence risks is dependent on an accurate diagnosis of the affected individual. Facial clefting, congenital heart disease, and neural tube defects can also be features of a large number of genetic syndromes, single gene disorders, chromosomal abnormalities, or the result of toxic effects from a maternal disease state or teratogen exposure. For these latter possibilities, it is suspected that such environmental factors lower the threshold for expression of susceptibility genes, rather than being the exclusive cause for the malformation.

A family history and detailed information about affected individuals should be obtained with specific inquiries about other, possibly mild, malformations and developmental problems. This information may suggest a specific syndrome and could significantly alter counseling about recurrence risks. For example, this woman should be examined for or questioned about the presence of lip pits. Lip pits are located on the lower lip and may appear as a pit or a mound of tissue. There may be a sinus tract that drains mucus. These pits are often removed surgically. The association of lip pits and cleft lip with or without cleft palate is seen in van der Woude syndrome, an autosomal dominant disorder.

Table 3.3 Empiric recurrence risk estimates (in percentages) for isolated orofacial clefts, neural tube defects and congenital heart defects

Affected family member	Neural tube defect*	Congenital heart defect**	Cleft lip $+/-$ cleft palate	Cleft palate
One sibling	2%	2–3%	1.2–5.1%	2%–5%
Two siblings	12%	10%	9–14%	10%–20%
Parent (sex not specified)	4%			3%–7%
Mother		5–6%	1.9–6.8%	
Father		2–3%	2–4.5%	
Aunt or uncle (second-degree relative)	1%	1–2%	0.4–0.8%	
First cousin (third-degree relative)	0.5%		0.2–0.5%	

*Assumes population incidence of 1/1000.
**Assumes population incidence of 1/200; percentages represent average risks for all types of congenital heart disease; recurrence risk for specific defects varies slightly around the above risk estimate.
From: Harper PS (2004) *Practical Genetic Counseling*, 6th edition. Oxford University Press, New York; Rimoin DL, Connor MJ, Pyeritz, RE *et al.* (2007) *Emery and Rimoin's Principles and Practice of Medical Genetics*, 5th edition. Reproduced with permission from Oxford University Press.

Published empiric data about the risk of recurrence of common multifactorial disorders can be reliably used for counseling purposes. Empiric data about the risk of recurrence in second-degree relatives are often not available or less precise. There are ethnic and geographic variations in the incidence of some multifactorial disorders, reflecting different genetic and/or environmental influences, which in turn may influence the risk of recurrence. Published data about recurrence risks for multifactorial disorders may be population-specific, with higher or lower recurrences being possible in other population groups or geographic areas.

Folate deficiency, which could be due to genetic variants affecting folic acid metabolism, the use of folic acid antagonists, or nutritional deficiencies, is now recognized as playing an important role in the pathogenesis of some multifactorial disorders such as facial clefting, neural tube defects, and congenital heart disease in some susceptible individuals.

Periconceptional folic acid supplementation has been shown to reduce the recurrence and occurrence risk of neural tube defects, facial clefting, and congenital heart disease. The recommendation for primary prevention of first occurrences of these and other malformations in women of reproductive age is folic acid supplementation at 0.4 mg per day. When a first-degree relative (i.e., sibling or parent) has a neural tube defect, the recommendation for prevention of a recurrence is 4 mg of folic acid per day, starting at least one month before becoming pregnant and continuing through the first few months of pregnancy. There are no known adverse effects on the fetus or mother of using folic acid supplementation for this period of treatment although a possible harmful effect of high dose folic acid has not yet

been excluded. There are no precise recommendations for folic acid prophylaxis for the prevention of recurrence of facial clefts and congenital heart disease or for pregnancies at increased risk for neural tube defects based on maternal medication use or a family history of an affected second-degree relative. Some practitioners recommend 4 mg per day and others suggest a lower dose.

Physical examination is unremarkable on the mother. The recurrence risk for cleft lip and palate based on empiric data (Table 3.3) is 2–7%. The risk for spina bifida is about 1% (affected second-degree relative), and the risk for a congenital heart disease is not increased over the general population risk.

Further reading

1 Czeizel AE, Dudas I (1992) Prevention of the first occurrence of neural-tube defects by periconceptional vitamin supplementation. *New England Journal of Medicine* 327:1832–1835.
2 Goldmuntz E, Woyciechowski S, Renstrom D *et al.* (2008) Variants of folate metabolism genes and the risk of conotruncal cardiac defects. *Circulation: Cardiovascular Genetics* 1:126–132.
3 Harper PS (2004) *Practical Genetic Counseling*, 6th edition. Oxford University Press, New York.
4 Hernandez-Diaz S, Werler MM, Walker, AM *et al.* (2000) Folic acid antagonists during pregnancy and the risk of birth defects. *New England Journal of Medicine* 343:1608–1614.
5 Holmes LB (1985) Malformations attributed to multifactorial inheritance. *Pediatrics in Review* 6:269–272.

6 Ionescu-Ittu R, Marelli AJ, Mackie AS *et al.* (2009) Prevalence of severe congenital heart disease after folic acid fortification of grain products: time trend analysis in Quebec, Canada. *BMJ* **338**:1673.

7 Rimoin DL, Connor MJ, Pyeritz RE *et al.* (2007) *Emery and Rimoin's Principles and Practice of Medical Genetics*, 5th edition.

8 Smith DA, Young IK, Refsum H (2008) Is folic acid good for everyone? *American Journal of Clinical Nutrition.* **87**:517–533.

9 Wilcox AJ, Lie RT, Solvoll K *et al.* (2007) Folic acid supplements and risk of facial clefts: national population case-control study. *BMJ* **334**(7591):464.

Autism

A couple is seen for genetics consultation following a psychological evaluation of their 3-year-old son who has been diagnosed with severe autistic spectrum disorder and mental retardation. The mother reports that she is 6 weeks pregnant and hopes to have prenatal diagnosis to look for a recurrence of her son's problems as his behavioral symptoms have overwhelmed the family.

Severe autism is one end of the autistic spectrum disorder which is characterized by varying degrees of abnormal and characteristic behavioral traits, and deficits in communication and social interaction. A number of lines of evidence show that genetic factors play an important role in the etiology of autism including a high concordance rate in monozygotic twins, a preponderance of affected males even at the milder end of the disease spectrum, and a recurrence risk in siblings which is much higher than the general population risk of occurrence.

Despite the evidence supporting high heritability for autism, the genetics of autistic spectrum disorder is complex and is poorly understood. An underlying genetic abnormality is found in only 6–15% of individuals despite extensive diagnostic evaluations. In addition to the large number of cytogenetic abnormalities detectable by routine metaphase analysis or array comparative genomic hybridization, at least 16 metabolic syndromes have been reported in association with an autism phenotype in which no structural birth defects are present. Autistic spectrum disorder has also been reported as an occasional feature of a large number of genetic syndromes (Table 3.4).

Because the underlying basis for the son's problems is unknown, risk of recurrence of a child with autistic spectrum disorder, which could be of greater or lesser severity than seen in the couple's son, is about 7%. (When the affected child is female, recurrence in a subsequent sibling is about 4%.) If two children are affected, the risk of recurrence approaches 50%.

The son has macrocephaly with a head circumference that is greater than 99ᵗʰ centile and postaxial polydactyly that was surgically corrected in infancy.

Anatomic abnormalities in association with autistic spectrum disorder increase the probability of a recognizable genetic syndrome.

In addition to the macrocephaly and scarring related to his postaxial polydactyly repair, physical examination of the

Table 3.4 Partial list of genetic syndromes with a reported association with autism

Fragile X syndrome
Apert syndrome
Rett syndrome
Williams syndrome
Angelman syndrome
De Lange syndrome
Prader–Willi syndrome
Noonan syndrome
Smith–Lemli–Opitz syndrome
Down syndrome
Smith–Magenis syndrome
Turner syndrome
Tuberous sclerosis
Neurofibromatosis
CHARGE syndrome
Myotonic dystrophy
Duchenne dystrophy
22q11 deletion syndrome
Moebius anomalad
Sotos syndrome
Cohen syndrome
PTEN associated disorders (Cowden syndrome, Bannayan–Riley–Ruvalcaba syndrome)
Oculo-auriculo-vertebral spectrum
Hypomelanosis of Ito
Joubert syndrome
Lujan–Fryns syndrome

Reproduced from: Schaefer GB, Mendelsohn NJ (2008) *Genetics in Medicine* **10**(1):4–12. Reproduced with permission from Lippincott, Williams & Wilkins.

son by a clinical geneticist reveals multiple papillomatous lesions around his mouth and nose. A family history is collected. No other relatives have autistic spectrum disorder. The couple's 5-year-old daughter is developmentally normal. The father's medical history is remarkable for a thyroidectomy for follicular thyroid cancer diagnosed at age 38 years. Physical examination of the father, who is of normal intelligence and has normal social interactions, shows papillomatous lesions on his face and macrocephaly. His mother died of uterine cancer.

The son with autistic spectrum disorder has the characteristic findings of Cowden syndrome, an autosomal dominant disorder caused by mutations in the *PTEN* gene. The *PTEN* gene is a tumor suppressor gene which regulates the ability of cells to proliferate and undergo apoptosis. In addition to Cowden syndrome, germ line mutations in the *PTEN* gene have been implicated in three other clinically distinct proliferative disorders, Bannayan-

Riley-Ruvalcaba syndrome, Proteus syndrome, and Proteus-like syndrome, all of which have some phenotypic overlap. Somatic *PTEN* mutations are present in many tumor types.

Common manifestations of Cowden syndrome include characteristic papillomatous skin lesions, a high risk of benign and malignant tumors most commonly affecting the thyroid, breast, and endometrium, and less frequently the kidney, mental retardation with autistic spectrum disorder, and macrocephaly. There is a wide range of severity and clinical findings in Cowden syndrome, even among members of the same family. Mutations in the *PTEN* gene causing Cowden syndrome are completely penetrant; by the third decade of life, virtually all individuals with a Cowden syndrome-related *PTEN* gene mutation will have at least the dermatologic manifestations of the disorder.

Molecular analysis of the son shows that he is heterozygous for a mutation in one of his PTEN genes. The mutation is subsequently documented in the father.

Other family members are at risk for having inherited the *PTEN* mutation. The father should be encouraged to inform his relatives of his diagnosis and the availability of clinical genetics evaluations and confirmatory molecular testing. Being forewarned about the increased risk of malignancies will allow for careful surveillance beginning at a relatively young age as directed by published oncology screening guidelines. Because the father's mother died of endometrial cancer, she is also likely to have been affected by Cowden syndrome. However, unless other maternal relatives have obvious signs of Cowden syndrome, the possibility of the mutation having been transmitted from his father, who died at a young age in an accident, should

not be discounted. Clinical evaluations of relatives from both the maternal and paternal sides of the father's family may be necessary.

Since the pathogenic mutation in the *PTEN* gene has been identified in the family, definitive prenatal diagnosis is available by chorionic villus sampling or amniocentesis, and preimplantation genetic diagnosis would be available for a future pregnancy. The fetus has a 50% risk of inheriting his father's *PTEN* gene mutation. About 12% of individuals with Cowden syndrome also have mental retardation. However, there are no data to allow predictions about the likelihood of a recurrence of an affected child who also has autistic spectrum disorder.

Further reading

1 Butler MG, Dasouki MJ, Zhou XP *et al.* (2005) Subset of individuals with autism spectrum disorders and extreme macrocephaly associated with germline PTEN tumour suppressor gene mutations. *Journal of Medical Genetics* **42**:318–321.

2 Eng C (2003) PTEN: one gene, many syndromes. *Human Mutation* **22**(3):183–198.

3 Eng C (Updated May 2009) *PTEN* Hamartoma Tumor Syndrome (PHTS). In *GeneReviews* at GeneTests: Medical Genetics Information Resource (database online). Copyright, University of Washington, Seattle. 1997–2009. Available at http://www.genetests.org. Accessed September 2009.

4 Muhle R, Trentacoste SV, Rapin I (2004) The genetics of autism. *Pediatrics* **113**(5):e472–486.

5 Schaefer GB, Mendelsohn NJ (2008) Genetics evaluation for the etiologic diagnosis of autism spectrum disorders. *Genetics in Medicine* **10**(1):4–12.

First and Second Trimester Screening

Historical overview

The utility of maternal serum biochemistry in providing information about the risk of fetal birth defects was first recognized in the late 1970s with the observation that maternal serum alpha-fetoprotein (AFP) at 15–20 weeks' gestation was usually elevated in the setting of a fetus with open spina bifida or an open ventral wall defect. By the mid-1980s, the association between fetal Down syndrome and decreased maternal serum AFP concentration (about 0.75 multiples of the normal median) led to widespread serum screening for Down syndrome in the early mid-trimester of pregnancy. Using maternal serum AFP concentration at 15–20 weeks' gestation and maternal age, 25% of Down syndrome-affected pregnancies in women under 35 years of age could be ascertained with a 5% false-positive rate. The incorporation into the screening paradigm of other serum markers followed shortly.

The combination of serum AFP, human chorionic gonadotropin (hCG), unconjugated estriol, and inhibin A (the "quadruple screen") and maternal age were incorporated into a statistical algorithm that allowed the detection of about two-thirds of Down syndrome pregnancies with a 5% false-positive rate. By the early 2000s, first trimester screening using the nuchal translucency measurement and hCG and PAPP-A in maternal serum between 11 and 14 weeks' gestation had largely supplanted second trimester screening for Down syndrome in some parts of the United States. This screening has

higher sensitivity (85–90%) and specificity (3% false-positive rate) for the detection of Down syndrome and is performed at an earlier gestational age. Integrated risk assessment at 16 weeks' gestation, which uses the nuchal translucency measurement and PAPP-A measurement from the first trimester and serum AFP, hCG, unconjugated estriol, and inhibin A from the second trimester, provides the highest sensitivity (93% detection rate) and specificity (3% false-positive rate) of screening tests in common use at the present time (2009).

In addition to providing information about the risks of Down syndrome and trisomies 13 and 18, screening in the first trimester occasionally will identify chromosomally normal fetuses with structural birth defects or genetic syndromes associated with an increased nuchal translucency. In the second trimester, markedly elevated serum AFP concentrations or very low unconjugated estriol concentrations will occasional identify rare maternal disease states or less common fetal abnormalities as illustrated by the following cases.

Increased nuchal translucency and a normal fetal karyotype

A 33-year-old woman was referred for first trimester screening. The nuchal translucency measurement obtained at 12 weeks' gestation was markedly increased at 6.2 mm (normal range: <3.5 mm). Because the risk of fetal

Prenatal Diagnosis: Cases & Clinical Challenges, 1st edition.   By Miriam S. DiMaio, Joyce E. Fox, Maurice J. Mahoney
Published 2010 by Blackwell Publishing Ltd.

aneuploidy was about 50% based on the increased nuchal translucency measurement, the patient elected to have chorionic villus sampling. The fetal karyotype was 46,XY.

Even in the presence of a normal fetal karyotype, an increased nuchal translucency measurement, present only in the first trimester, is associated with an increased risk for a large number of genetic syndromes and major structural birth defects (Table 4.1). Many are very rare. The risk of fetal anomalies is directly correlated with the magnitude of the nuchal translucency measurement. A heart defect is the most common birth defect observed. The risk of congenital heart disease is about 3% for nuchal translucency measurements between 3.5 and 4.5 mm, and is 30% for a nuchal translucency measurement of 6.5 mm or more. Skeletal dysplasias, as a group, are the next most common fetal abnormality. Many, but not all, of the fetal abnormalities associated with an increased nuchal translucency measurement can be identified by further prenatal testing.

Detailed ultrasonographic examination should be performed at 16–18 weeks' gestation to evaluate the fetal anatomy and to assess whether the nuchal measurement is in the normal range or is persistently increased. A persistently increased or enlarging nuchal measurement would be associated with a high risk of underlying fetal pathology. Another detailed ultrasonographic examination and fetal echocardiography should be performed at 20–22 weeks' gestation.

If the increased nuchal translucency measurement in the first trimester resolves over the next few weeks and the fetus continues to appear normal by sonography, which includes fetal echocardiography at 20–22 weeks' gestation, the most likely outcome of the pregnancy will be a normal baby. However, there remains a small chance of underlying fetal pathology of varying severity that will not be evident by prenatal sonography.

In the patient's pregnancy, detailed ultrasonographic examination at 16 weeks' gestation revealed normal-appearing fetal anatomy and fetal growth. Fetal echocardiography at 22 weeks' gestation revealed Tetralogy of Fallot.

The absence of other fetal abnormalities on ultrasound examination suggests that the heart defect is isolated. However, an underlying syndrome associated with congenital heart disease remains a possibility. Congenital heart defects are commonly seen in the 22q11 microdeletion syndrome (also known as DiGeorge syndrome or velocardiofacial syndrome). This syndrome has variable intrafamilial expression and is often associated with congenital heart disease and other abnormalities including thymic (T cell) immune deficiency, hypoparathyroidism, dysmorphic facies, palatal abnormalities including clefts, learning disabilities, mild mental retardation, seizures, autism, schizophrenia, bipolar disorder, and renal dysplasia. About 15% of individuals with Tetralogy of Fallot also have a chromosome 22q11 microdeletion.

In the setting of congenital heart disease, with or without an increased nuchal translucency measurement in the first trimester, fluorescence in situ hybridization (FISH) analysis using a probe for the chromosome 22q11 microdeletion or array comparative genomic hybridization should be offered.

In this patient's pregnancy, FISH analysis revealed the presence of the chromosome 22q11 microdeletion. Predictions about the severity of problems associated with the microdeletion syndrome are not possible although some assessment of the presence and severity of T-cell deficiency could be addressed with a fetal blood sample.

Risk of recurrence of the chromosome 22q11 microdeletion syndrome in a future pregnancy depends on whether the microdeletion arose de novo (which occurs in 93% of cases), or whether it was inherited from an affected parent who had unrecognized features of the disorder. Therefore, FISH analysis of parents' peripheral blood cell chromosomes for the chromosome 22q11 microdeletion is indicated. If one of the parents has the microdeletion, risk of recurrence in a future pregnancy would be 50% although predictions about the severity of expression of the disorder would not be possible. If neither parent has evidence of the microdeletion in their peripheral blood chromosomes, risk of recurrence would be very small, less than 1%, but increased over the general background risk. This small increased risk reflects the possibility of gonadal mosaicism for the microdeletion in one of the parents.

Had fetal echocardiography revealed normal-appearing fetal anatomy, the yield of further molecular testing to investigate a genetic basis of the increased nuchal translucency measurement is small. It is currently not feasible to perform molecular analysis of genes for multiple different disorders because the incidence of each disorder and the detection rate for disease-causing mutations are small. Array comparative genomic hybridization to look for gene deletions and duplications undetectable by routine chromosomal analysis would

Table 4.1 Abnormalities identified in fetuses with first-trimester increased nuchal translucency measurements

Central nervous system defect	*Skeletal defect*	*Facial defect*
Acrania/anencephaly	Achondrogenesis	Agnathia/micrognathia
Agenesis of the corpus callosum	Achondroplasia	Facial cleft
Craniosynostosis	Asphyxiating thoracic dystrophy	Microphthalmia
Dandy–Walker malformation	Blomstrand osteochondrodysplasia	Treacher–Collins syndrome
Diastematomyelia	Campomelic dysplasia	
Encephalocele	Cleidocranial dysplasia	*Fetal anemia*
Fowler syndrome	Hypochondroplasia	Blackfan Diamond anemia
Holoprosencephaly	Hypophosphatasia	Congenital erythropoietic porphyria
Hydrolethalus syndrome	Jarcho–Levin syndrome	Dyserythropoietic anemia
Iniencephaly	Kyphoscoliosis	Fanconi anemia
Joubert syndrome	Limb reduction defect	Parvovirus B19 infection
Macrocephaly	Nance–Sweeney syndrome	Alpha thalassemia
Microcephaly	Osteogenesis imperfecta	
Spina bifida	Roberts syndrome	*Nuchal defect*
Trigonocephaly C	Robinow syndrome	Cystic hygroma
Ventriculomegaly	Short rib polydactyly syndrome	Neck lipoma
Sirenomelia	Talipes equinovarus	
	Thanatophoric dwarfism	*Pulmonary defect*
Cardiac defect	VACTERL association	Cystic adenomatoid malformation
Ventricular septal defect		Diaphragmatic hernia
Atrioventricular septal defect	*Neuromuscular defect*	Fryns syndrome
Hypoplastic left heart	Fetal akinesia deformation sequence	
Tetralogy of Fallot	Myotonic dystrophy	*Metabolic defect*
Pulmonary stenosis	Spinal muscular atrophy	GM1 gangliosidosis
Wolff–Parkinson–White syndrome		LCHAD
	Gastrointestinal defect	Mucopolysaccharidoses
Abdominal wall defect	Crohn disease	Smith-Lemli-Opitz syndrome
Cloacal exstrophy	Duodenal atresia	Vitamin D resistant rickets
Exomphalos	Esophageal atresia	Zellweger syndrome
Gastroschisis	Small bowel obstruction	
Other defect	*Genitourinary defect*	
Body stalk anomaly	Ambiguous genitalia	
Brachmann-de Lange syndrome	Congenital adrenal hyperplasia	
CHARGE syndrome	Congenital nephrotic syndrome	
Deficiency of the immune system	Hydronephrosis	
Congenital lymphedema	Hypospadias	
EEC syndrome	Infantile polycystic kidneys	
Neonatal myoclonic encephalopathy	Meckel–Gruber syndrome	
Noonan syndrome	Megacystis	
Perlman syndrome	Multicystic dysplastic kidneys	
Stickler syndrome	Renal agenesis	

Reproduced from Souka AP, Von Kaisenberg CS, Hyett JA *et al.* (2005) *American Journal of Obstetrics and Gynecology* **192**:1005–1021. Reproduced with permission from Elsevier.

have a low yield as most of the genetic disorders known to be associated with a first trimester increased nuchal translucency measurement are caused by point mutations. Case reports suggest that Noonan syndrome may have a significant probability when the fetal phenotype in the second trimester includes pleural effusions or hydrops fetalis. Testing for at least some of the associated genes can be performed.

Markedly elevated serum AFP concentration unexplained by a fetal defect on ultrasound

A 27-year-old woman is referred because of a serum AFP concentration that is 8.7 multiples of the median. A detailed ultrasonographic examination performed at 18 weeks' gestation reveals normal-appearing fetal anatomy. In the hands of an experienced sonologist and with optimal visualization of the fetus, 90–95% of open neural tube defects and the majority of ventral wall defects should be identifiable by prenatal sonography.

The differential diagnosis of a markedly elevated serum AFP concentration which is unexplained by a fetal defect apparent on ultrasonographic examination includes the following.

1 *Placental pathology* is the most likely explanation for the markedly elevated serum AFP concentration. It may represent a fetal-maternal bleed at the uterine-placental interface. This is not a rare occurrence and usually is a transient and isolated event.

Placental abnormalities such as chorioangiomas, placental lakes, and inflammatory disease allow increased transudation of fetal proteins into the maternal circulation. Elevated maternal serum AFP levels in the absence of fetal abnormalities are associated with an approximate threefold increased risk of stillbirth, preterm delivery, and intrauterine growth restriction. In association with an elevated hCG concentration determined at the time of quadruple or integrated risk assessment, the increased risk is six- to sevenfold.

Some maternal autoimmune disease states such as systemic lupus erythematosis can be associated with autoantibodies that can lead to decidual vasculopathy and an elevated serum AFP concentration.

2 *Fetal disease* Some very rare defects of the fetal kidneys and skin can cause leakage of fetal proteins but not be detectable by ultrasonographic examination. One of these is congenital nephrosis, often termed Finnish-type congenital nephrosis, which is a rare autosomal recessive disorder; renal transplantation is often necessary for effective treatment. Disorders of the skin are of variable severity and include cutis aplasia, large hemangiomas, and epidermolysis bullosa. Epidermolysis bullosa is a group of disorders which are characterized by varying degrees of skin fragility and recurrent blister formation. The most severe forms have autosomal recessive inheritance and are often fatal early in life due to severe epithelial blistering of the respiratory, digestive, and genitourinary systems, in addition to skin involvement.

There remains a small chance of an open body defect (i.e., neural tube or ventral wall defect) undetected by ultrasonographic examination. There are also rare reports of families with hereditary persistence of elevated concentrations of AFP.

3 *Maternal disease states* such as hepatitis, hepatoma, or metastatic or toxic liver disease may also account for the elevated serum AFP concentration.

When the maternal serum AFP concentration is mildly elevated (between 2–3 multiples of the median), the likelihood that the concentration of AFP in amniotic fluid will help to identify a fetal defect is small. Whether to proceed with amniocentesis is debatable in this circumstance and should consider the skills of the sonologist, the risk of amniocentesis, patient preferences, and economic considerations.

However, when the serum AFP is moderately or markedly elevated as illustrated by this case, the risks of underlying fetal pathology undetectable by ultrasonographic examination become greater and amniocentesis for measurement of amniotic fluid AFP should be given serious consideration.

Elevated amniotic fluid AFP concentration

If the amniotic fluid AFP concentration is elevated, this suggests that the fetus is leaking excessive AFP. An alternative explanation would be a placental defect that is allowing leakage of fetal proteins into the amniotic fluid space.

When the amniotic fluid AFP concentration is elevated, further testing should include testing for acetylcholinesterase. Acetylcholinesterase will be present in the setting of neural tube defects and lesions in which neural tissue is exposed. It may not be present in the setting of a ventral wall defect. It would be present in the setting of a severe denuding skin disorder such as epidermolysis bullosa but may not be present for other skin defects. The acetylcholinesterase will be absent in the setting of congenital nephrosis.

Both denuding skin disorders and congenital nephrosis are very rare conditions. It is important to recognize that congenital nephrosis does not occur exclusively among people of Finnish ancestry where the incidence is about 1.2 per 10 000 births. In the United States the incidence of congenital nephrosis is estimated at 1 in 50 000. An estimated 1 out of every 150 000 live births is affected with some type of epidermolysis bullosa. The severe denuding form of autosomal recessive epidermolysis bullosa has an incidence of about 0.5 per million live births.

Providing probability estimates about the likelihood of either of these disorders or other fetal pathology with an unexplained amniotic fluid AFP elevation is inexact. Decisions about further diagnostic testing should take into account the extent of the AFP elevation in amniotic fluid and the presence or absence of acetylcholinesterase.

Congenital nephrosis is genetically heterogeneous; mutations in at least four genes have been associated with congenital nephrosis. Gene sequencing of the *NPHS1* gene will identify a high percentage of disease-causing mutations among individuals of Finnish ancestry. However, for individuals of other ancestral backgrounds, the overall sensitivity in detecting disease-causing mutations in the *NPHS1* or other congenital nephrosis-associated genes is unknown. In the absence of a family history, gene sequencing may not have utility in the prenatal setting given the low chance of an affected fetus, the unknown mutation detection rate, and the length of time required for molecular analysis. Elevated amniotic fluid albumin levels have been reported in some, but not all, affected pregnancies.

Prenatal diagnosis of epidermolysis bullosa can be accomplished by fetal skin biopsy and examination of the skin by electron microscopy. Fetal skin biopsy is associated with up to 3% risk of miscarriage and an additional few percent risk of extreme prematurity, and is performed in only a few centers nationwide. Sequencing of multiple recessively inherited epidermolysis bullosa-associated genes will find about 95% of mutations when performed in individuals who are affected. In this prenatal scenario, the chance of epidermolysis bullosa is small, and the time frame required for molecular analysis is usually several weeks, which is suboptimal when gestational age is advanced and decisions about pregnancy termination must be made quickly. As developments in gene chip technology and gene sequencing advance, testing for common mutations causing severe epidermolysis bullosa and congenital nephrosis should become faster and less expensive.

Normal amniotic fluid AFP concentration

When the amniotic fluid AFP concentration is normal, a fetal source of the elevated protein concentration seen in maternal serum is very unlikely. This leaves a placental process which is allowing more AFP to transudate into the maternal circulation or a maternal disease state as possible explanations. Sometimes placental abnormalities (e.g., chorioangiomas) are visible on ultrasonographic examination but most often the placenta has a normal appearance.

Maternal disease states such as hepatitis or a hepatic malignancy are rare explanations for an elevated serum AFP concentration during pregnancy. A careful medical history and drug/medication exposure history should be collected. For example, the serum AFP concentration can be elevated with acute liver injury due to acetaminophen toxicity.

When an initial serum AFP determination is ≥ 5 multiples of the median, a second serum AFP determination should be obtained a few weeks after the initial result to determine whether it continues to rise or is falling. A falling concentration will provide reassurance that a maternal disease state is unlikely. A significant rise in AFP concentration should initiate an evaluation of the mother which would include liver function tests and ultrasonographic imaging of the maternal abdomen. Consultation with other specialists might also be indicated. Amniocentesis can cause transient elevations of serum AFP; therefore, waiting two weeks following amniocentesis for the repeat determination is recommended.

Very low or undetectable concentration of unconjugated estriol

The serum uE_3 concentration is virtually undetectable in the serum sample of a 26-year-old woman at second trimester ("quadruple") screening. The serum AFP, hCG, and inhibin A concentrations are unremarkable. A detailed ultrasonographic examination at 18 weeks' gestation reveals normal-appearing fetal anatomy and growth.

The differential diagnosis of a very low serum uE_3 concentration (<0.2 ng/mL or <0.15 multiples of the median) includes the following:

1 *Non-pregnant state*: a woman who is not pregnant will have a very low uE_3 concentration.

2 A pregnancy at *less advanced date* than presumed by the laboratory will have a low uE_3 concentration reported because the concentration of unconjugated estriol increases in maternal serum during the second trimester.

3 *Intrauterine fetal death* is a common explanation for a very low serum uE_3 concentration.

4 *Fetal pathology* can be the explanation.
- Chromosomal abnormalities such as triploidy, trisomy 18, or Down syndrome can be associated with a very low uE_3 concentration.
- Steroid (placental) sulfatase deficiency associated with X-linked ichthyosis may be present. Steroid sulfatase deficiency is the most common explanation for a

very low serum uE_3 concentration when the fetus is alive and pregnancy dating is correct. The clinical findings include scaly, dry skin. Steroid sulfatase deficiency is usually of mild or moderate degree and does not have effects on intelligence or longevity. The disorder is commonly mistaken for excessively "dry skin" and is underdiagnosed.

When the fetus is male and has normal-appearing anatomy as determined by ultrasonographic examination, a very low serum uE_3 is associated with a significant risk of X-linked ichthyosis (steroid sulfatase deficiency) whether or not a family history of the disorder is present. The gene is on the short arm of the X chromosome (Xp22.32). A large majority of mutations are gene deletions. A family history of male relatives with excessively dry, scaly, or eczematous skin is frequently elicited.

Deletions at Xp22 are associated with ichthyosis and, if they extend beyond the steroid sulfatase gene, with other findings such as mental retardation, hypogonadism, chondrodysplasia punctata, and Kallmann syndrome (anosmia/hyposmia, decreased intelligence, abnormal movements and other neurologic findings, and occasional heart and kidney abnormalities). The risk of such an expanded ichthyosis phenotype is small (a few percent).

• Smith–Lemli–Opitz syndrome is an autosomal recessive disorder of cholesterol biosynthesis with an estimated incidence ranging from 1 in 10 000 to 1 in 40 000. It is the second most common explanation for a low maternal serum uE_3 concentration in viable fetuses with correct pregnancy dating. Affected individuals have elevated levels of 7-dehydrocholesterol due to a deficiency of 7-dehydrocholesterol reductase and may have hypocholesterolemia.

Smith–Lemli–Opitz syndrome has a wide clinical spectrum which, at the severe end, is typically associated with prenatal and postnatal growth retardation, ambiguous genitalia in males, microcephaly, moderate to severe mental retardation, cleft palate, and multiple major and minor malformations. Some affected individuals have only mild symptoms that would not be detectable by prenatal sonography. Intrauterine fetal death may occur for the most severely affected individuals. Maternal serum uE_3 concentrations in affected pregnancies range from undetectable to 0.65 multiples of the median, with a median of 0.23 multiples of the median. Using a cut-off of 0.15 multiples of the median (equivalent to a risk cut-off of 1 in 50) will detect about 60% of affected pregnancies; 1 in 300

pregnancies will have a positive screen result at this cut-off (Palomaki *et al.* 2002).

• Multiple sulfatase deficiency is a rare and usually fatal autosomal recessive neurodegenerative disorder of infancy and early childhood. It is due to absence of arylsulfatases A, B, and C; arylsulfatase C is steroid sulfatase. Coarsened facial features, bony abnormalities, and ichthyosis are present, plus increased tissue deposition of acid mucopolysaccharides.

• Adrenal hypoplasia or aplasia is included in the differential diagnosis of a very low serum uE_3 concentration. Adrenal hypoplasia/aplasia can be due to a primary adrenal defect; X-linked and autosomal recessive disorders have been reported. Alternatively, hypoplasia of the adrenal glands can be secondary to pituitary or hypothalamic developmental defects, or to structural defects of the central nervous system disrupting pituitary or hypothalamic function. A major structural defect in the brain would be unlikely if intracranial anatomy appears normal by ultrasonographic examination.

• A number of rare enzyme deficiencies in pathways of steroidogenesis can result in a low serum uE_3 concentration, which include: 20,22 desmolase deficiency; 17-alpha hydroxylase deficiency; 3-beta-OH dehydrogenase deficiency; 17,20 desmolase deficiency; blocks in testosterone to estrogen conversion.

In the setting of a very low uE_3 concentration determined as part of quadruple screening, the following should be accomplished.

First, the report of biochemical serum screening should be reviewed to verify whether the correct gestational age was used to calculate the multiples of the median for uE_3 and the other serum analytes. A pregnancy that is significantly less advanced than used in the risk calculation could be associated with a report of very low serum uE_3 concentration. Verification of the patient's last menstrual period, the regularity of her menstrual cycle, and review of any early dating ultrasonographic examinations will aid in establishing whether the correct gestational age was used in calculating the results of biochemical serum screening.

Detailed ultrasonographic examination should be performed to evaluate the fetal anatomy. The fetal sex and the presence and appearance of the adrenal glands should be noted. Low uE_3 concentrations are often associated with an increased risk for both Down syndrome and trisomies 18 and 13 so that amniocentesis is often offered to establish the fetal karyotype.

After the viability and correct dating of the pregnancy have been confirmed, a careful family history should be collected including queries about male relatives with dry or scaly skin.

If the fetus is male, X-linked ichthyosis due to steroid sulfatase deficiency is by far the most common pathologic explanation for a low serum estriol concentration. Available data suggest that more than half of normal boys born to women with low unconjugated estriol concentration are subsequently diagnosed with ichthyosis or other chronic skin disorders such as eczema or seborrheic dermatitis, with the latter two diagnoses possibly representing a misdiagnosis. A surprising number of patients describe brothers, fathers, maternal grandfathers or maternal uncles or other male relatives with dry or scaly skin for which an underlying cause has never been established. The absence of such a family history does not exclude the diagnosis. New mutations of the steroid sulfatase gene will also occur in some families.

FISH analysis can be performed on amniotic fluid cells to look for common deletions on the X chromosome associated with steroid sulfatase deficiency. This analysis could also be performed on the patient's peripheral blood chromosomes if invasive testing is not elected and the family history raises suspicions for the disorder. Additional probes or array CGH methods can look for contiguous gene deletions.

After steroid sulfatase deficiency, the next most likely fetal abnormality that could be associated with a low maternal serum uE_3 is Smith–Lemli–Opitz syndrome. The prenatal diagnosis of this syndrome is accomplished by measurement of 7-dehydrocholesterol in amniotic fluid supernatant or chorionic villus cells. DNA analysis would also be possible if the disease-causing mutations have been identified. This latter approach is useful in families who have had a previous affected child and are seeking early diagnosis of Smith–Lemli–Opitz syndrome. Identification of disease-causing mutations usually takes several weeks and is not practical when concerns about Smith–Lemli–Opitz syndrome have been raised for the first time by a low maternal serum uE_3 concentration. Maternal serum and urine steroid analysis as a non-invasive diagnostic alternative to amniotic fluid steroid analysis is also showing promise in the diagnosis of Smith–Lemli–Opitz syndrome in high-risk pregnancies. The diagnosis of steroid sulfatase deficiency can also be made by measurement of maternal urine steroids.

There are major limitations to addressing other entities in the above differential diagnosis. All are rare disorders so the a priori risks are small, even with the low serum uE_3. Enzyme testing is not available and mutation testing of known genes is not practical at present. If the results of testing for steroid sulfatase deficiency and Smith–Lemli–Opitz syndrome are normal, the most likely outcome of the pregnancy will be normal. However, there remains a small chance of underlying fetal disease associated with the abnormally low serum uE_3.

Further reading

1 Crandall BF, Matsumoto M (1991) Risks associated with an elevated amniotic fluid alpha fetoprotein level. *American Journal of Medical Genetics* **39**:64–67.

2 Crandall BF, Matsumoto M (1986) Routine amniotic fluid alpha fetoprotein assay: experience with 40,000 pregnancies. *American Journal of Medical Genetics* **24**:143–149.

3 Palomaki GE, Bradley LA, Knight GJ *et al.* (2002) Assigning risk for Smith-Lemli-Opitz syndrome as part of 2nd trimester screening for Down's syndrome. *Journal of Medical Screening* **9**:43–44.

4 Pfendner E, Lucky A (Updated 10/2007) Dystrophic Epidermolysis Bullosa. In: *GeneReviews* at GeneTests: Medical Genetics Information Resource (database online). Copyright, University of Washington, Seattle. 1997–2009. Available at http://www.genetests.org. Accessed September 2009.

5 Schoen E, Norem C, O'Keefe J *et al.* (2003) Maternal serum unconjugated estriol as a predictor for Smith–Lemli–Opitz syndrome and other fetal conditions. *Obstetrics and Gynecology* **102**:167–172.

6 Senat MV, Bussières L, Couderc S *et al.* (2007) Long-term outcome of children born after a first-trimester measurement of nuchal translucency at the 99th percentile or greater with normal karyotype: a prospective study. *American Journal of Obstetrics and Gynecology* **196**:53.e1–6.

7 Shackleton CH, Marcos J, Palomaki GE *et al.* (2007) Dehydrosteroid measurement in maternal urine or serum for the prenatal diagnosis of Smith Lemli Opitz syndrome (SLOS). *American Journal of Medical Genetics Part A* **143A**:2129–2136.

8 Souka AP, Von Kaisenberg CS, Hyett JA *et al.* (2005) Increased nuchal translucency with normal karyotype. *American Journal of Obstetrics and Gynecology* **192**:1005–1021.

Abnormal Ultrasound Findings

Recurrent hypotonia and polyhydramnios

A 30-year-old woman is seen for consultation during her sixth pregnancy at 8 weeks' gestation. Her first pregnancy resulted in the birth of a healthy boy. All subsequent pregnancies were complicated by severe fetal hypotonia and polyhydramnios in the second or third trimester of pregnancy. Club feet were noted in two of the pregnancies. One of the pregnancies resulted in a term stillbirth. The others were electively terminated at about 23 weeks' gestation. Three were female; one was male. Physical examination of the fetuses revealed joint contractures. Pathological examinations were uninformative; no structural abnormalities were noted. In particular, no pterygium (webbing) of the joints was seen. Karyotypes were established for three of the affected fetuses and were normal.

The findings in the affected fetuses are consistent with the fetal akinesia deformation sequence, a condition in which multiple joint contractures (arthrogryposis multiplex congenita) are present due to decreased intrauterine fetal movement. Fetal akinesia deformation sequence is an etiologically heterogeneous condition. Causes include underlying abnormalities of the central or peripheral nervous system, of muscle, of connective tissue, intrauterine vascular compromise, maternal disease states, and space constraints within the womb. Although the majority of cases are associated with low recurrence risk, some cases of fetal akinesia deformation sequence are due to an underlying chromosomal abnormality or mutations in a gene coding

for inherited disorders with autosomal dominant, autosomal recessive, X-linked, or mitochondrial inheritance.

Either an inherited disorder or a maternal disease state has a high probability of explaining the patient's obstetric history. Among the inherited disorders, autosomal recessive and autosomal dominant conditions need to be considered. X-linked inheritance is very unlikely given that three of the affected babies were female. Mitochondrial inheritance with a mildly affected mother should also be considered although such disorders are very rare.

A number of different autosomal recessive disorders must be considered. The probability that a couple would have four of five pregnancies affected by an autosomal recessive condition is about 1 in 68; the probability that they would have the pregnancies in the order in which they occurred, first one normal and then four affected, is 1 in 341. The absence of birth defects and pterygia is an important clue because most autosomal recessive disorders associated with fetal akinesia usually have other findings in addition to decreased fetal movement. Spinal muscular atrophy due to mutations in the *SMN1* gene would be the most common autosomal recessive condition. *SMN1* gene analysis could be performed on an affected fetus or the parents. Although an autosomal recessive disorder cannot be excluded, other causes should be considered.

A detailed family history and a physical examination of the mother should be performed. Maternal myotonic dystrophy or myasthenia gravis could explain the woman's pregnancy history.

Prenatal Diagnosis: Cases & Clinical Challenges, 1st edition.   By Miriam S. DiMaio, Joyce E. Fox, Maurice J. Mahoney
Published 2010 by Blackwell Publishing Ltd.

Myotonic dystrophy is an autosomal dominant disorder with highly variable expression which includes progressive muscle weakness, myotonia, cardiac conduction defects, cataract formation, and endocrine abnormalities. Mutations in at least two different genes can cause myotonic dystrophy. Mutations in the *DMPK* (dystrophia myotonia-protein kinase) gene result in DM1, the most common form of the disorder. It is a CTG trinucleotide expansion disorder in which repeat sizes of $\geq$50 CTG repeats within the gene are associated with expression of the disorder. The severity and age of onset of the clinical manifestations are generally correlated with the size of the trinucleotide expansion. In addition, a large CTG repeat is susceptible to considerable expansion when transmitted by an affected mother. Very large CTG repeat expansions are associated with the severe congenital form of the disorder in which hypotonia and respiratory insufficiency are present that sometimes are lethal in the neonatal period. Of those who survive the neonatal period, mental retardation is present in 50–60%. Polyhydramnios and decreased fetal movement are often present prenatally in the congenital form. At the other end of the clinical spectrum, mildly affected individuals may go unrecognized and have a normal lifespan. Occasionally, a woman may be found to have mild symptoms of myotonic dystrophy only after the birth of a child with the severe congenital form. The chance that a woman with myotonic dystrophy would have four of five pregnancies, in any order, in which the fetus inherited her abnormal *DM1* gene is about 16%, although the probability of transmission *and* expansion to the congenital form would be smaller.

Another maternal disease state that could result in severe fetal hypotonia is myasthenia gravis which is an autoimmune neuromuscular disease resulting in varying degrees of muscle weakness. It is caused by the production of autoantibodies against human acetylcholine receptors. Affected women have an increased risk of pregnancy loss, prematurity, and maternal mortality and morbidity. In addition, transplacental passage of the antibodies results in neonatal myasthenia gravis in 10–20% of children born to affected mothers. Neonatal myasthenia gravis usually results in transient respiratory and feeding difficulties. It is a rare cause of arthrogryposis multiplex congenita.

A family history is collected. The patient's father had cataract surgery at age 52 years. At age 60 years, he was diagnosed with diabetes. The patient's paternal uncle required a pacemaker at age 55 years. Both the father and uncle are bald. The patient's physical examination was remarkable for sustained muscle contractions when asked to shake the examiner's hand. She had evidence of mild facial muscle weakness. Ophthalmologic evaluation revealed the presence of bilateral posterior subcapsular cataracts. She had no functional disability.

The presence of findings typical of myotonic dystrophy in the patient and subtle signs of the disorder in her father and paternal uncle suggest that her fetal losses were caused by the congenital form of myotonic dystrophy. Molecular testing of the patient shows that she has a CTG repeat size of 420 repeats in one of her *DMPK* genes, compatible with the findings of mild myotonic dystrophy. Transmission of this gene is associated with a significant risk of CTG expansion in her children. Analysis of DNA saved from one of the affected fetuses identified a CTG repeat size of 2200 repeats, consistent with the diagnosis of congenital myotonic dystrophy. Women with 100 or more CTG repeats in one of their *DMPK* genes have over 60% chance of transmitting a gene to their child that has expanded into the range which causes congenital myotonic dystrophy. The earlier age of onset and increased severity of myotonic dystrophy in each succeeding generation illustrates the phenomenon of anticipation which is due to the instability of the enlarged CTG repeat during female transmission. A similar phenomenon occurs in the transmission of enlarged fragile X alleles (premutation alleles) from women or Huntington disease alleles from men.

Prenatal diagnosis of the *DMPK* gene size is now possible for this patient in her current pregnancy by chorionic villus sampling or amniocentesis. Preimplantation genetic diagnosis would also be available in future pregnancies.

Further reading

1 Bird TD (Updated November 2007) Myotonic Dystrophy Type I. In: *GeneReviews* at GeneTests: Medical Genetics Information Resource (database online). Copyright, University of Washington, Seattle. 1997–2009. Available at http://www.genetests.org. Accessed September 2009.

2 Cobo AM, Poza JJ, Martorell L *et al.* (1995) Contribution of molecular analyses to the estimation of the risk of congenital myotonic dystrophy. *Journal of Medical Genetics* 32:105–108.

3 Redman JB, Fenwick RG Jr, Fu YH *et al.* (1993) Relationship between parental trinucleotide GCT (sic) repeat length and severity of myotonic dystrophy in offspring. *Journal of the American Medical Association* 269(15):1960–1965.

Holoproscencephaly

A 24-year-old woman is referred for genetic counseling because a previous pregnancy with her current partner was complicated by an ultrasonographic examination at 22 weeks' gestation which revealed alobar holoprosencephaly. The pregnancy was terminated by induction of labor; pathologic examination of the fetus after delivery confirmed the diagnosis of alobar holoprosencephaly; no other anatomic defects were identified. The fetal karyotype, obtained via amniocentesis at the time of pregnancy termination, was normal (46,XY). The woman and her partner have unremarkable family histories. The woman is obese and has poorly controlled type 2 insulin-dependent diabetes.

Holoprosencephaly is etiologically heterogeneous and has genetic and environmental causes. Maternal diabetes is a known risk factor for fetal holoprosencephaly conferring a 200-fold increased risk. Animal models suggest that in utero exposure to teratogenic agents such as alcohol, retinoic acid, and cholesterol-lowering medications may also be associated with an increased risk.

Holoprosencephaly can be a feature of chromosomal abnormalities. Trisomy 13, trisomy 18, triploidy, and a number of different structural chromosomal abnormalities account for between 25 and 50% of cases of holoprosencephaly.

Holoprosencephaly is an occasional feature of at least 25 syndromic genetic disorders in which other anatomic problems are also present and which are associated with autosomal recessive or autosomal dominant inheritance. For example, an infrequent cause of holoprosencephaly is Smith–Lemli–Opitz syndrome, a disorder of cholesterol biosynthesis, which will usually be accompanied by a decreased maternal serum unconjugated estriol concentration.

Mutations in at least 15 different genes are known or thought to cause non-syndromic holoprosencephaly (i.e., holoprosencephaly without other birth defects). These include cases in which the disorder can be transmitted to a baby from a very mildly affected parent via a mutation in an autosomal dominant gene. Although it is unlikely that either the woman or her husband would have mild features of holoprosencephaly, it is advisable that they both be examined by an experienced medical geneticist. Occasionally a parent has a single central maxillary incisor or ocular hypotelorism, which is their only manifestation of an autosomal dominant mutation, resulting in a severe phenotype in their child. The highly variable phenotype among members of the same family who carry an autosomal dominant mutation causing holoprosencephaly presumably reflects the effects of other modifying genes and/or intrauterine or environmental factors which are not yet understood Most cases of non-syndromic holoprosencephaly arise due to new dominant mutations or de novo chromosomal abnormalities.

Submicroscopic gene deletions or duplications account for about 5% of cases of holoprosencephaly. Array comparative genomic hybridization (CGH) could be performed on fetal DNA if fetal tissue were available from the autopsy or if fetal DNA had been extracted and saved.

The couple has an evaluation by a clinical geneticist who finds no anatomic evidence of a microform of holoprosencephaly in either parent. Review of the results of the woman's quadruple screen from the affected pregnancy showed that the serum estriol concentration was normal (1.2 multiples of the median) which makes the diagnosis of Smith–Lemli–Opitz syndrome very unlikely. Array CGH of DNA obtained from frozen fetal tissue does not identify a chromosomal duplication or deletion.

In the absence of an identified cause, the empiric recurrence risk of holoprosencephaly is estimated at 4% which reflects the experience of most families in which the disorder does not recur and a few families in which there is high recurrence risk due to an underlying genetic syndrome which has Mendelian inheritance. Maternal diabetes is associated with a 1% chance of holoprosencephaly. Whether the woman's poorly controlled diabetes was the primary etiologic factor causing holoprosencephaly in her fetus cannot be proven but suggests that the risk of recurrence might be significant in a subsequent pregnancy if her diabetes is poorly controlled and there are other underlying susceptibility factors. Good diabetes management beginning prior to conception and continuing throughout gestation and careful surveillance of the fetus by ultrasonographic examination is indicated for a future pregnancy.

Further reading

1 Bendavid C, Dubourg C, Gicquel I *et al.* (2006) Molecular evaluation of foetuses with holoprosencephaly shows high incidence of microdeletions in the HPE genes. *Human Genetics* **119**(1–2):1–8.
2 Chen CP, Chen CY, Lin CY *et al.* (2005) Prenatal diagnosis of concomitant alobar holoprosencephaly

and caudal regression syndrome associated with maternal diabetes. *Prenatal Diagnosis* **25**(3):264–266.

3 Heussler HS, Suri M, Young ID *et al.* (2002) Extreme variability of expression of a Sonic Hedgehog mutation: attention difficulties and holoprosencephaly. *Archives of Disease in Childhood* **86**:293–296.

4 Kelley RL, Roessler E, Hennekam RC *et al.* (1996) Holoprosencephaly in RSH/Smith-Lemli-Opitz syndrome: does abnormal cholesterol metabolism affect the function of Sonic Hedgehog? *American Journal of Medical Genetics* **66**(4):478–484.

5 Muenke M, Gropman A (Updated 3/5/2008) Holoproscencephaly. In: *GeneReviews* at GeneTests: Medical Genetics Information Resource (database online). Copyright, University of Washington, Seattle. 1997–2009. Available at http://www.genetests.org. Accessed September 2009.

6 Nanni L, Schelper RL, Muenke MT (2000) Molecular genetics of holoprosencephaly. *Frontiers in Bioscience* **5**: D334–342.

Abnormalities of the digits

Ultrasonographic examination performed at 21 weeks' gestation reveals that both feet of a fetus have absence deformities. The right foot appears to have a single digit and probable absence of four metatarsals; the metatarsals are probably present in the left foot but only three central digits are present. All other fetal anatomy appeared normal including the tibial lengths.

Amniotic rupture sequence might account for the fetal defects. However, the abnormalities could readily have a genetic etiology. The defects are bilateral and affect the distal lower limbs.

Online Mendelian Inheritance in Man (OMIM) lists 55 syndromes in which absent digits are a feature. Most genetic entities, however, involve abnormalities of both the hands and the feet. Abnormalities of other organ systems may also be present including the central nervous system (microcephaly, seizures, mental retardation), the kidneys, skin, face (clefts), hearing, genitalia, eyes, and long bones. Most of the genetic syndromes have autosomal dominant inheritance. A few with autosomal recessive or X-linked inheritance are also described.

Future sonographic imaging of the fetus including magnetic resonance imaging (MRI) is unlikely to provide more information about the presence of other birth defects. A three-dimensional ultrasonographic examination might provide better resolution of the face and feet

and perhaps give more insight into the possibility of amniotic bands as the etiology of the fetal abnormalities. Endoscopy to better view the fetus is also unlikely to yield definitive information and entails significant risk.

There is only a small probability that a karyotypic abnormality is the underlying cause of the fetal abnormalities. However, if a chromosomal abnormality is present, the chance of central nervous system and other organ system involvement would be high. There is no molecular testing available to address the possibility of a Mendelian disorder.

Examination of the parents is indicated to look for evidence of subtle skeletal abnormalities.

After delivery, consultation with a clinical geneticist is indicated to obtain a specific diagnosis and information about prognosis and recurrence.

Multicystic kidneys

Ultrasonographic examination performed at 18 weeks' gestation in a 25-year-old primigravida revealed enlarged echogenic kidneys containing multiple small cysts and moderately decreased amniotic fluid volume. Another ultrasonographic examination performed at 20 weeks' gestation confirmed the renal findings and showed worsening oligohydramnios.

The prenatal diagnosis of renal cysts raises a large differential diagnosis. Achieving a correct diagnosis of the fetus prior to delivery is often difficult but is critical for accurate counseling about prognosis and risk of recurrence.

Unilateral or bilateral multicystic dysplastic kidney disease (MCDKD) is the most frequent renal abnormality encountered on prenatal ultrasonographic examination with an incidence of 1 in 1000 to 1 in 5000 births. It is usually sporadic, with low risk of recurrence, and most often arises due to an obstructive process during renal development. The kidneys may be hypoplastic or enlarged. In part this depends on the nature of the abnormal developmental process. It will also depend on the location of the obstruction, i.e., is it due to ureteral atresia at the ureteropelvic junction or due to a lower urinary tract obstruction (e.g., posterior urethral valves)?

Familial recurrences of MCDKD without other abnormalities have also been reported. In these families, the recurrence may be due to an autosomal dominant gene with decreased penetrance and variable expressivity or multifactorial inheritance. Either can result in the situation where a parent with undiagnosed unilateral

Table 5.1 Examples of genetic syndromes associated with prenatally diagnosed cystic kidney disease

Chromosomal
  Trisomy 13
  Trisomy 18
Autosomal recessive
  Ellis–van Creveld syndrome
  Fryns syndrome
  Infantile polycystic kidney disease
  Jeune asphyxiating thoracic dystrophy
  Joubert syndrome
  Marden–Walker syndrome
  McKusick–Kaufman syndrome
  Robert syndrome
  Short rib polydactyly syndromes
  Smith–Lemli–Opitz syndrome
  Zellweger syndrome
X-linked
  Oro-facial-digital syndrome (X-linked dominant)
  Simpson–Golabi–Behmel syndrome (X-linked recessive)
Autosomal dominant
  Autosomal dominant polycystic kidney disease
   (adult polycystic kidney disease)
  Tuberous sclerosis
  Townes–Brock syndrome
  Alagille syndrome
  Renal coloboma syndrome
  Cystic dysplasia with *TCF2* mutations

Reproduced from Sanders RC (2002) *Structural Fetal Abnormalities*, 2nd edition. Mosby, St Louis MO. London with permission of Elsevier LTD.

multicystic kidney has a child with unilateral or bilateral disease diagnosed in utero.

MCDKD can be a feature of a large number of genetic syndromes (Table 5.1). Most are rare and would often be associated with other manifestations visible on prenatal ultrasonographic examination. In addition, maternal diabetes and maternal rubella infection, maternal exposure to thalidomide and ACE inhibitors, and fetal hypoxia have all been linked to an increased risk of MCDKD.

Heterozygous mutations in the *TCF2* (transcription factor 2) gene are an important cause of bilateral hyperechogenic kidneys and kidneys with cystic dysplasia. The phenotype associated with *TCF2* gene mutations is highly variable, even among members of the same family. Extrarenal findings may be present and include urogenital abnormalities and maturity-onset diabetes of the young.

Autosomal dominant polycystic kidney disease (PKD) is one of the most common multisystem genetic disorders among adults with an incidence of about 1 in 800. Almost all affected individuals have a mutation in one of two genes, *PKD1* or *PKD2*, which account for 85% and 15% of cases, respectively. Clinical onset of kidney disease is usually between 30 and 50 years but can vary widely among affected individuals in the same family. Cases with prenatal onset of renal findings identifiable by ultrasonographic examination occur rarely. Prenatal findings include enlarged kidneys, hyperechogenic renal cortex and medulla, and diminished or absent corticomedullary differentiation. Small bilateral cortical cysts may or may not be present. Amniotic fluid volume is normal. In rare families, unilateral renal hypoplasia or aplasia has been reported.

Occasionally the diagnosis of autosomal dominant PKD is first made in a fetus or in a young child who has a presymptomatic parent. Also, about 5% of cases are due to de novo mutations in *PKD1* or *PKD2* genes. In the absence of a family history of the disorder, autosomal dominant polycystic kidney disease has only a small chance of being the cause of echogenic cystic kidneys.

Autosomal recessive polycystic kidney disease (infantile polycystic kidney disease) is a rare disorder occurring in 1 in 20 000 to 1 in 50 000 births. There is a wide range of interfamilial and intrafamilial phenotypic severity and age of onset. Fifty percent of cases are identifiable by prenatal ultrasonography. Kidneys can be grossly enlarged resulting in a large abdominal circumference with echogenic renal parenchyma and loss of corticomedullary differentiation. However, renal cysts are not evident in the first or second trimester in most prenatally diagnosed cases. Amniotic fluid volume ranges from normal to absent.

Mutations in one gene, *PKHD1* (polycystic kidney and hepatic disease 1), cause autosomal recessive polycystic kidney disease. There is no evidence for a second locus.

In order to maximize the chance of a establishing a diagnosis for the fetus, further prenatal testing should include documentation of the presence or absence of extrarenal abnormalities by prenatal ultrasonographic examination and renal ultrasonographic examinations for both parents. Fetal chromosome analysis can be obtained by chorionic villus sampling if severe oligohydramnios is present, or by bladder puncture for urinary tract cells if the bladder is distended. After delivery, the baby should have a careful examination by a nephrologist. If the baby does not survive, a complete pathologic examination of the fetus is indicated. In addition, DNA should be obtained from fetal tissue for possible molecular diagnostic testing in the future.

Further reading

1 Aubertin G, Cripps S, Coleman G *et al.* (2002) Prenatal diagnosis of apparently isolated unilateral multicystic kidney: implications for counselling and management. *Prenatal Diagnosis* **22**:388–394.

2 Bisceglia M, Galliani CA, Senger C *et al.* (2006) Renal cystic diseases: a review. *Advances in Anatomic Pathology* **13**:26–56.

3 Decramer S, Parant O, Beaufils S *et al.* (2007) Anomalies of the TCF2 gene are the main cause of fetal bilateral hyperechogenic kidneys. *Journal of the American Society of Nephrology* **18**:923–933.

4 Harris P, Rossetti S (2004) Molecular genetics of autosomal recessive polycystic kidney disease. *Molecular Genetics and Metabolism* **81**:75–85.

5 Pei Y (2003) Molecular genetics of autosomal dominant polycystic kidney disease. *Clinical and Investigative Medicine* **26**:252–258.

6 Winyard P, Chitty L (2001) Dysplastic and polycystic kidneys: diagnosis, associations and management. *Prenatal Diagnosis* **21**:924–935.

Omphalocele

Ultrasonographic examination performed at 17 weeks in a 37-year-old woman due to an elevated serum AFP concentration revealed a fetal omphalocele. Fetal growth and all other fetal anatomy appeared normal. Amniocentesis revealed a normal female karyotype. Fetal echocardiography at 22 weeks' gestation was also normal. The pregnancy was conceived via in vitro fertilization due to several years of unexplained infertility. Both parents have normal peripheral blood karyotypes and the husband has normal sperm parameters. First trimester screening predicted low risks for Down syndrome and trisomies 18 and 13.

Omphalocele can occur as an isolated abnormality or as one feature of a number of Mendelian and chromosomal disorders (Table 5.2).

In about two-thirds of cases of omphalocele, there are associated malformations including heart defects, neural tube defects, facial clefting, diaphragmatic hernia, bladder extrophy, and imperforate anus. With the exception of imperforate anus, most of these abnormalities should be evident on prenatal ultrasonographic examination.

When omphalocele is the only finding on ultrasonographic examination and the fetal karyotype is normal, there still remains a several percent risk of a genetic syndrome although an isolated omphalocele remains the most likely

Table 5.2 Disorders in which omphalocele is a feature

Chromosomal abnormalities
Trisomy 13
Trisomy 18
Down syndrome
Triploidy
Syndromes
Amniotic band syndrome
Beckwith–Wiedemann syndrome
Carpenter syndrome
CHARGE association
Meckel–Gruber syndrome
Pentalogy of Cantrell
Valproate teratogenicity
Short rib polydactyly syndromes

Reproduced from Sanders RC (2002) *Structural Fetal Abnormalities*, 2nd edition. Mosby, St Louis MO; London reproduced with permission from Elsevier.

outcome. Of the possible genetic syndromes which could be present, Beckwith–Wiedemann syndrome (BWS) would be the most likely with an estimated chance of 5–20%.

BWS is a generalized somatic overgrowth disorder whose typical features may include macrosomia, abdominal wall defects, ear creases, ear pits, and neonatal hypoglycemia. There is also an increased risk for embryonal tumors, hemihypertrophy, and visceromegaly of various tissues and organs. A number of different genetic mechanisms can lead to BWS including: (1) imprinting defects affecting gene methylation at the *BWS* locus on chromosome 11p15; (2) segmental uniparental disomy at the *BWS* gene locus; and (3) chromosomal abnormalities involving the *BWS* locus.

Imprinting defects in one or both of the *BWS* gene clusters on one chromosome 11p15 are the most common cause of BWS. Abnormal methylation of maternally inherited genes in this region results in abnormal transcription of one or more genes which regulate cell growth and accounts for 50–60% of cases of BWS. In 20% of cases, there is paternal uniparental disomy at the *BWS* locus which results functionally in absence of the maternally inherited genes at the *BWS* locus. In BWS, paternal uniparental disomy is segmental (i.e., involves only a small portion of chromosome 11p including the *BWS* gene cluster), rather than whole chromosome uniparental disomy. One to two percent of cases of BWS are the result of a cytogenetic abnormality such as a translocation, inversion, or duplication which results in disruption of imprinted gene expression. In families with de novo cases of BWS, 5–10% are due to mutations in the *CDKN1C* gene which is also part of the *BWS* gene domain. Some phenotypic predictions with respect to the probability of childhood malignancy can be made depending on which *BWS* gene cluster contains the molecular alteration.

Prenatal testing to investigate the possibility of BWS in a fetus with an omphalocele and no other abnormalities can be done sequentially. Routine cytogenetic analysis of amniotic fluid or chorionic villus cells to look for cytogenetic abnormalities would be an initial step in investigating an omphalocele. Only rarely would BWS be accompanied by cytogenetic abnormalities so fetal DNA should be obtained from the cells for possible molecular analysis. If the fetal karyotype is normal, uniparental disomy studies looking for evidence of paternal uniparental disomy and methylation studies to look for other imprinting defects can be accomplished by molecular analysis of DNA obtained from the prenatal specimen and the parents' leukocytes. This approach could lead to the prenatal diagnosis of about 75% of fetuses with BWS who have an omphalocele as the only feature of the disorder.

Sequencing of the fetal *CDKN1C* genes to identify mutations is not widely available and may not be feasible to accomplish in a timely way to help with decisions about pregnancy management. If the diagnosis of BWS is confirmed after delivery, gene sequencing should be performed if other molecular explanations have not been found.

Analysis of DNA obtained from cultured amniocytes and the parents' leukocytes shows abnormal maternal methylation at the BWS gene locus, confirming the diagnosis of BWS in the fetus. The parents wonder whether there is a connection between the disorder and their use of assisted reproductive technology (ART).

Studies have suggested that there is a sixfold increased risk of BWS among the offspring of pregnancies conceived via ART. Furthermore, of 24 reported cases of BWS which have occurred in ART-conceived pregnancies, 23 were due to maternal methylation defects where only 50–60% of all cases of BWS are expected to have an underlying methylation abnormality. There are also reports of an excess of ART-conceived children with Angelman syndrome due to a maternal imprinting defect. This information suggests that, in some embryos, ART may adversely affect normal gene imprinting. A competing hypothesis is that some characteristic of one or both of the parents that is associated with their infertility might be the basis for an increased risk of an imprinting disorder. By this hypothesis, ART would circumvent effective biological mechanisms that would normally prevent conception and thus result in improved fitness of individuals predisposed to having children with genetic disorders.

Further reading

1 Halliday J, Oke K, Breheny S *et al.* (2004) Beckwith-Wiedemann syndrome and IVF: a case-control study. *American Journal of Human Genetics* **75**:526–528.
2 Li M, Squire JA, Weksberg R (1998) Molecular genetics of Wiedemann-Beckwith syndrome. *American Journal of Medical Genetics* **79**:253–259.
3 Sanders RC (2002) *Structural Fetal Abnormalities*, 2nd edition. Mosby, St Louis MO; London.
4 Weksberg R, Shuman C, Beckwith JB (2010) Beckwith-Wiedemann syndrome. *European Journal of Human Genetics* **18**:8–14.
5 Wilkins-Haug L, Porter, A, Hawley P *et al.* (2009) Isolated fetal omphalocele, Beckwith–Wiedemann syndrome, and assisted reproductive technologies. *Birth Defects Research (Part A): Clinical and Molecular Teratology* **85**:58–62.
6 Williams DH, Gauthier DW, Maizels M (2005) Prenatal diagnosis of Beckwith–Wiedemann syndrome. *Prenatal Diagnosis* **25**:879–884.

Recurrent fetal hydrops

A healthy 31-year-old presents for genetic counseling early in her fifth pregnancy. Her first pregnancy resulted in the birth of a healthy boy. In her second and third pregnancies, severe fetal hydrops developed between 18 and 20 weeks' gestation. Both fetuses, a male and female, had normal karyotypes. Pathologic examination of the second hydropic fetus and placenta and electron microscopy of chorionic villi did not reveal any abnormalities. The woman's fourth pregnancy resulted in the term birth of a boy who had severe neonatal thrombocytopenia (platelet count 6000 per microliter). He was treated with intravenous immunoglobulin, had a good response to therapy, and is developing normally. Platelet antigen genotyping of the woman and her husband shows that the woman is homozygous for PLA2 and the husband is homozygous for PLA1.

This woman's three most recent pregnancies have been complicated by recurrent, severe fetal hydrops or alloimmune thrombocytopenia.

Prior to the 1960s, Rh isoimmunization was the leading cause of hydrops fetalis. The advent of Rh immune globulin has led to a dramatic reduction in hydrops fetalis due to fetal Rh disease and a consequent rise in the proportion of cases which have a non-immune basis. There are a large number of conditions which have been reported in association with fetal hydrops (see Table 5.3).

These include structural malformations of the heart, kidneys, liver and genitourinary tract, cardiac arrhythmias, vascular and lymphatic malformations, chromosomal abnormalities, single gene disorders including a number of lysosomal storage disorders, fetal neoplasms,

Table 5.3 Conditions associated with non-immune hydrops

Cardiovascular

Malformation
  Left heart hypoplasia
  Atrioventricular canal defect
  Right heart hypoplasia
  Closure of foramen ovale
  Single ventricle
  Transposition of the great arteries
  Ventricular septal defect
  Atrial septal defect
  Tetralogy of Fallot
  Ebstein's anomaly
  Premature closure of ductus
  Truncus arteriosus
  Aortic or pulmonary stenosis
  Valvular insufficiency
Tachyarrhythmia
  Atrial flutter
  Paroxysmal atrial tachycardia
  Wolff–Parkinson–White
  Supraventricular tachycardia
Bradyarrhythmia including complete
  heart block
Other arrhythmia
High-output failure
  Neuroblastoma
  Sacrococcygeal teratoma
  Large fetal angioma
  Placental chorioangioma
  Umbilical cord hemangioma
Cardiac tumors
Other cardiac neoplasia
Cardiomyopathy
Cardiosplenic syndromes

Chromosomal

45, X
Trisomy 21
Trisomy 18
Trisomy 13
18q +
13q −
45, X/46, XX
Triploidy

Chondrodysplasias

Thanatophoric dwarfism
Short rib polydactyly
Hypophosphatasia
Osteogenesis imperfecta
Achondrogenesis

Twin pregnancy

Twin-twin transfusion syndrome
Acardiac twin

Hematologic

Alpha-thalassemia
Fetomaternal transfusion
Parvovirus B19 infection
In utero hemorrhage
Glucose-6-phosphatedehydrogenase
  (G6PD) deficiency
Red cell enzyme deficiencies
Thrombosis of major vessels
Leukemia
Red cell aplasias

Thoracic

Congenital cystic adenomatoid
  malformation of lung
Diaphragmatic hernia
Intrathoracic mass
Pulmonary sequestration
Chylothorax
Airway obstruction
Pulmonary lymphangiectasia
Pulmonary neoplasia
Bronchogenic cyst

Infections

Cytomegalovirus (CMV)
Toxoplasmosis
Parvovirus B19 (fifth disease)
Syphilis
Herpes
Rubella
Coxsackievirus
Leptospirosis

Malformation sequences and genetic syndromes

Congenital lymphendema, e.g., Noonan's syndrome
Arthrogryposis
Multiple pterygia
Neu–Laxova syndrome
Pena–Shokeir syndrome
Myotonic dystrophy
Saldino–Noonan syndrome
Francois syndrome, type III

Metabolic

Gaucher's disease
GM$_1$ gangliosidosis
Sialidosis
Hurler syndrome
Mucopolysaccharide (MPS) IVa
Mucolipidosis type I + II
Pyruvate kinase deficiency
Galactosialidosis

Urinary Tract

Urethral stenosis or atresia
Posterior urethral valves
Congenital nephrosis (Finnish type)
Prune belly syndrome

Gastrointestinal

Midgut volvulus
Malrotation of the intestines
Duplication of the intestinal tract
Meconium peritonitis
Hepatic fibrosis
Cholestasis
Biliary atresia
Hepatic vascular malformations
Hepatitis
Hepatic necrosis
Liver tumors or cysts

infections, maternal disease states, and exposure to drugs or medications. These diverse etiologies reflect the equally diverse underlying mechanisms which have been postulated to lead to fetal hydrops including abnormalities of lymphatic drainage in the thoracic and abdominal cavities, increased capillary permeability, increased venous pressure, and reduced osmotic pressure.

Among infectious causes, infection with parvovirus B19 is the most common cause of fetal hydrops and accounts for 25–30% of cases in otherwise anatomically normal fetuses. Parvovirus infections between 10 and 20 weeks' gestation are associated with the highest risk of fetal damage.

This occurs primarily because of interference with the normal development of red cell precursors leading to severe anemia in the setting of an expanding blood volume. The virus may also infect the myocardium leading to myocarditis and high-output cardiac failure. After the diagnosis of the first affected fetus, parvovirus B19 and TORCH (toxoplasma, rubella, cytomegalovirus, herpes simplex virus) infections were explored by maternal serology which did not show evidence of a recently acquired infection. After the diagnosis of a second affected pregnancy, the likelihood of a fetal infection became very small.

Even after the exclusion of major fetal malformations, chromosomal abnormalities, common maternal infections and exposures, and maternal disease states, the lack of feasibility of testing for the large number of single gene disorders associated with fetal hydrops often precludes a diagnosis.

Prior to the birth of her son with alloimmune thrombocytopenia, the cause of the hydrops remained elusive. Autosomal recessive inheritance would seem to have been the most likely explanation for her affected pregnancies although it is possible that either the woman or her husband could have germline mosaicism for a dominantly inherited condition. An unrecognized immune-mediated disorder is also a possibility and should be given greater consideration once the woman was subsequently discovered to be sensitized to fetal platelet antigens.

Because the woman is homozygous for *PLA2* antigens and her husband is homozygous for *PLA1*, all offspring of the couple will be PLA1/PLA2 heterozygotes. No fetal testing is necessary to establish the fetal genotype. In each of her pregnancies, the fetus is at risk for the complications of alloimmune thrombocytopenia, which usually develop in utero but may also occur in the immediate newborn period. While most affected fetuses do not suffer complications, intracranial hemorrhage of variable severity leading to an abnormal neurologic outcome occurs in utero in 20–30% of cases. In women who are sensitized to fetal platelet antigens, the expected situation would be increasing severity of fetal alloimmune thrombocytopenia with each successive pregnancy because of a more robust maternal immune response, although some children with alloimmune thrombocytopenia with clinical sequelae are born to primiparous women.

The couple's platelet incompatibility might be etiologically related to the fetal hydrops. However, there are only a few reports in the literature of fetuses affected with both conditions who have had other common causes of fetal hydrops excluded.

Khouzami and colleagues have proposed several mechanisms which could associate fetal hydrops with alloimmune thrombocytopenia. These include a severe fetal hemorrhage leading to either severe anemia or cardiac insufficiency, or hepatic dysfunction due to increasing extramedullary hepatic hematopoiesis which leads to obstructed portal venous blood flow, portal hypertension and ascites. Decreased fetal albumin production leading to hypoalbuminemia and generalized edema may also occur in the setting of hepatocellular damage.

Treatment of the woman with intravenous immunoglobulin +/− corticosteroids and careful monitoring of the pregnancy has been shown to decrease the likelihood of potentially devastating fetal complications of alloimmune thrombocytopenia. The woman should be managed by a specialist in maternal fetal medicine.

Further reading

1 Burin MG, Scholz AP, Gus R et al. (2004) Investigation of lysosomal storage diseases in nonimmune hydrops fetalis. *Prenatal Diagnosis* **24**(8):653–657.

2 Khouzami AN, Kickler TS, Callan NA et al. (1996) Devastating sequelae of alloimmune thrombocytopenia: an entity that deserves more attention. *Journal of Maternal Fetal Medicine* **5**:137–141.

3 Kooper AJ, Janssens PM, de Groot AN et al. (2006) Lysosomal storage diseases in non-immune hydrops fetalis pregnancies. *Clinica Chimica Acta* **371** (1–2):176–182.

4 Lockwood CJ, Julien S (2009) Non-immune hydrops fetalis. *Up To Date on line*.

5 Paidas M (2009) Prenatal management of neonatal alloimmune thrombocytopenia. *Up To Date on line*.

6 von Kaisenberg CS, Jonat W (2001) Fetal parvovirus B19 infection. *Ultrasound in Obstetrics and Gynecology* **18**:280–288.

7 Williamson LM, Hackett G, Rennie J et al. (1998) The natural history of fetomaternal alloimmunization to the platelet-specific antigen HPA-1a (PlA1, Zwa) as determined by antenatal screening. *Blood* **92**:2280–2287.

Non-motile ciliopathies

A 22-year-old primiparous woman was referred for consultation due to an ultrasonographic examination performed at 28 weeks' gestation which revealed an encephalocele with evidence of brain herniation, massively enlarged fetal kidneys, a left rocker-bottom foot, and a right clubbed hand with postaxial polydactyly. The long bones and ribs appeared normal in shape and size. Fetal echocardiography was normal.

Given the severe abnormalities noted on ultrasonographic examination, prognosis for long-term survival of the fetus is poor, regardless of the underlying diagnosis. However, accurate counseling about recurrence risks and prenatal or preimplantation genetic diagnosis requires a diagnosis. The abnormal ultrasonographic findings could be explained by trisomy 13, another chromosomal abnormality, or by one of several single gene disorders.

An amniocentesis is performed and reveals a normal female karyotype and normal concentration of 7- dehydrocholesterol, excluding Smith–Lemli–Opitz syndrome.

Renal abnormalities, encephalocele, and postaxial polydactyly are features of Bardet–Biedl syndrome, Meckel–Gruber syndrome, and Joubert syndrome, all of which are rare autosomal recessive disorders. These abnormalities can also be seen in Jeune syndrome (asphyxiating thoracic dystrophy), another autosomal recessive disorder, but the fetus lacks the usual skeletal findings which include shortened limbs and a small narrow thorax due to shortened ribs.

The genetic diseases noted above are included in a class of disorders known as non-motile ciliopathies. This group of disorders is distinct from the primary ciliary dyskinesias which are disorders of motile beating cilia that affect the motility of sperm and respiratory tract cilia. The non-motile ciliopathies arise due to abnormalities of primary cilia whose function is involved in crucial developmental and physiologic cell signaling pathways, thus explaining the deleterious multisystem effects often seen in these disorders. The characteristic pathology that may be present in the non-motile ciliopathies includes cystic kidneys, liver disease, brain malformations, situs inversus, polydactyly, retinal degeneration, and skeletal defects as shown in Table 5.4. Other non-motile ciliopathies with different clinical presentations include autosomal recessive and autosomal dominant polycystic kidney disease, nephronophthisis, Senior–Loken syndrome, Alstrom syndrome, oro-facial-digital syndrome type I, Ellis–van Creveld syndrome, and Leber congenital amaurosis. More than 30 genes associated with ciliopathy syndromes have been identified.

All of these disorders are characterized by clinical manifestations that have a wide range of severity. They are also characterized by marked genetic heterogeneity in which mutations in a number of different loci lead to the same or similar clinical findings. For example, 15 genes are known to be associated with Bardet–Biedl syndrome, six genes are associated with Meckel–Gruber syndrome,

Table 5.4 Common clinical features of the ciliopathies

Feature	BBS	MKS	JBTS	NPHP	SLSN	JATD	OFD1	EVC	ALMS	PKD
Renal cysts	x	x	x	x	x	x	x			x
Hepatobiliary disease	x	x	x	x	x	x	x		x	x
Laterality defect	x	x		x		x				
Polydactyly	x	x	x			x	x	x		
Agenesis of corpus callosum	x	x	x			x	x			
Cognitive impairment	x	x	x			x	x	x		
Rentinal degeneration	x	x	x		x	x			x	
Posterior fossa defects/encephalocele	x	x	x			x		x		
Skeletal bone defects						x	x	x		
Obesity	x								x	

BBS, Bardet–Biedl syndrome; MKS, Meckel syndrome; JBTS, Joubert syndrome; NPHP, nephronophthisis; SLSN, Senior–Loken syndomre; JATD, Jeune syndrome; OFD1 oro-facial-digital syndrome type 1; EVC, Ellis–van Creveld syndrome; ALMS, Alstrom syndrome; PKD, polycystic kidney disease.
Reproduced from Tobin JI, Beales PL (2009) *Genetics in Medicine* **11**(6):386–402. Reproduced with permission from Lippincott, Williams & Wilkins.

eight genes are associated with Joubert syndrome and at least two genes are associated with both Jeune syndrome and Ellis–van Creveld syndrome.

To further complicate the picture, there is considerable phenotypic overlap between some of these disorders, and some of the non-motile ciliopathies with distinctly different clinical presentations are due to mutations in the same gene. In some cases of Bardet–Biedl syndrome triallelic inheritance may occur. This complex inheritance pattern occurs when three mutations are responsible for the disease (two mutations are present at one locus and a third mutation occurs at a second locus) Thus, non-motile ciliopathies that have clinical and genotypic overlap may not be distinct disorders but rather part of a phenotypic continuum which is influenced by the nature of the mutations that are present and, in some cases, the number of those mutations.

After delivery, pathologic examination of the fetus or infant may help narrow the diagnosis. Molecular testing to confirm a clinical diagnosis of one of the ciliopathies associated with multisystem abnormalities is currently available for only some of the disorders under consideration.

Even for the disorders in which molecular analysis is possible, testing at present is a major undertaking in an ongoing pregnancy because of the large number of genes associated with each disorder and the relatively small fraction of cases which are due to mutations in any one gene. Testing of all known disease-causing loci is not currently available on a clinical basis.

Future pregnancies are at 25% risk of recurrence and serial ultrasonographic examination beginning early in the pregnancy would probably find most affected fetuses. However, intrafamilial variability may result in a less severe phenotype that might not be detectable by fetal imaging.

Further reading

1 Baala L, Romano S, Khaddour R *et al.* (2007) The Meckel-Gruber Syndrome gene (MKS3) is mutated in Joubert Syndrome. *American Journal of Human Genetics* **80**(1):186–194.

2 Chen CP (2007) Meckel syndrome: genetics, perinatal findings, and differential diagnosis. *Taiwanese Journal of Obstetrics and Gynecology* **46**:9–14.

3 Consugar MB, Kubly VJ, Lager DJ *et al.* (2007) Molecular diagnostics of Meckel-Gruber syndrome highlights phenotypic differences between MKS1 and MKS3. *Human Genetics* **121**:591–599.

4 Katsanis N, Ansley SJ, Badano JL *et al.* (2001) Triallelic inheritance in Bardet-Biedl syndrome, a Mendelian recessive disorder. *Science* **293**:2256–2259.

5 Tobin JI, Beales PL (2009) The nonmotile ciliopathies. *Genetics in Medicine* **11**(6):386–402.

6 Common Issues in Prenatal Diagnosis

Prenatal Diagnosis: Cases & Clinical Challenges, 1st edition.   By Miriam S. DiMaio, Joyce E. Fox, Maurice J. Mahoney
Published 2010 by Blackwell Publishing Ltd.

Introduction to common issues in prenatal diagnosis

The topics in this chapter bring together common issues in genetic counseling and the delivery of prenatal diagnosis services such as the interpretation of family and medical histories, parental consanguinity, non-paternity, and infertility.

A core concept in genetic counseling is the collection of accurate and complete family and maternal histories, and the utilization of that information in the risk assessment of birth defects and genetic disorders. Accurate risk assessment is dependent upon a correct diagnosis. Errors in diagnosis and hence risk assessment may occur when genetic disorders with different patterns of inheritance have overlapping clinical presentations, or when a genetic disorder masquerades as a condition that is usually explained by multifactorial or environmental factors.

Consanguinity raises concerns about the risk of birth defects and genetic disorders. Assessment of the degree of relatedness of the parents is required to establish whether a consanguineous mating places a future child at increased risk for autosomal recessive and multifactorial conditions. The cultural aspects of consanguineous marriages, which are common in some parts of the world, are also important to consider.

Non-paternity may be inadvertently detected as a result of prenatal diagnosis and may complicate the interpretation of results. The discovery of non-paternity may raise ethical questions about the risks and benefits of disclosure to a patient and the impact of that information on the integrity of relationships among family members.

The widespread accessibility of assisted reproductive technologies has resulted in an increasing number of pregnancies conceived via in vitro fertilization and related procedures. Infertility or subfertility is the most common reason for use of these technologies, and in some instances the etiology may be unknown yet still due to an inherited cause. Utilization of assisted reproductive technologies may circumvent natural barriers to reproduction, resulting in the transmission of genetic abnormalities and an increased risk of birth defects and genetic disorders.

Infertility

Case 1 A healthy 27-year-old woman and her husband are referred for genetic counseling. She has no children and has had three first trimester miscarriages. Her family history includes a sister who had multiple congenital abnormalities and died in the neonatal period. No further information about this individual is available. Her mother also had an early miscarriage and a stillbirth at 35 weeks' gestation. The patient has two other sisters.

Around 10 to 15% of couples have fertility problems. Infertility, or early pregnancy loss that mimics infertility, can occur because of a balanced chromosomal rearrangement in one of the parents. Balanced chromosomal rearrangements, i.e., translocations and inversions, are found in a few percent of phenotypically normal individuals who have experienced recurrent spontaneous pregnancy loss. When a woman has had two or three miscarriages, chromosomal analysis of both members of the couple should be performed.

In this woman's situation, the information that she had a sibling with multiple birth defects further increases the chance that the woman carries a chromosomal rearrangement.

Chromosomal analysis of both members of the couple reveals that the woman has an apparently balanced reciprocal translocation [46,XX, t(3;18)(q28;q12.2)]. Her husband has a normal karyotype.

In this reciprocal translocation, a small segment of the long arm of chromosome 3 has exchanged locations with about three-quarters of the long arm of chromosome 18. Because the translocation has been identified in a healthy adult woman and no cytogenetic material is missing at this level of resolution, it is unlikely to have important health implications for her. Nonetheless, there is potential disruption of genes situated at or near the translocation breakpoints and this issue should be reviewed every few years as more information about these genes becomes available.

The reciprocal translocation results in the production of abnormal gametes which can lead to infertility, recurrent early loss of chromosomally unbalanced embryos, or viable unbalanced fetuses who can survive postnatally with significant functional and structural abnormalities. The likelihood of a viable unbalanced fetus depends, in part, on the size of the imbalance. Unbalanced transloca-

tions with large partial trisomies or monosomies are usually lost very early in gestation. Survival into later pregnancy or the neonatal period is more likely when small imbalances are present or when full trisomy for the chromosome involved in the translocation is compatible with long-term survival, as is the case for chromosome 18. In this woman's situation, her translocation places her at a significant risk for an unbalanced fetus who inherits three copies of part of the long arm of chromosome 18 and may survive into the second trimester or beyond. The pregnancy history of the woman's mother raises suspicions that she or the woman's father also carries the balanced translocation and that some chromosomally unbalanced fetuses may survive into late pregnancy or beyond.

Fetuses who inherit the woman's balanced translocation would be expected to be normal. However, there are circumstances in which two family members with the same translocation have different phenotypes due to a variety of reasons. These include the inheritance of two copies of a recessive gene whereas the parent had only a single copy, small duplications or deletions of genetic material at or close to the translocation breakpoints, and epigenetic phenomena as discussed in more detail in Chapter 1 in the section on reciprocal translocations and structural abnormalities.

Prenatal diagnosis with chorionic villus sampling or amniocentesis is one option for this couple. Preimplantation genetic diagnosis could be utilized to identify embryos with unbalanced translocations and introduce only chromosomally normal or balanced embryos to the womb. The woman's sisters and other at-risk relatives should be informed of their increased chance of carrying the chromosomal translocation.

Case 2 A non-consanguineous couple is referred for genetic counseling after a fertility evaluation revealed severe oligospermia. They are now considering in vitro fertilization and intracytoplasmic sperm injection. Both members of the couple are in their mid-thirties.

About 10 to 15% of couples have fertility problems. In about half of couples with infertility, sperm production is abnormal, either qualitatively or quantitatively; some of these men have an underlying genetic abnormality.

Intracytoplasmic sperm injection (ICSI) is the principal treatment for male factor infertility. Even in the setting of severe oligospermia or azoospermia, immature spermatozoa can be retrieved via an epididymal aspiration or testicular biopsy. Thus, ICSI circumvents effective biological mechanisms for sperm selection and improves the biological fitness of some men who have an underlying genetic abnormality.

The three most common genetic causes of male infertility are constitutional chromosomal abnormalities, microdeletions on the Y chromosome, and mutations in the cystic fibrosis (*CFTR*) gene located on chromosome 7. Less common explanations include androgen insensitivity, androgen receptor mutations, congenital adrenal hyperplasia, Kallmann syndrome, Noonan syndrome, and Kartagener syndrome and other primary ciliary dyskinesias.

In azoospermia and severe oligospermia an underlying constitutional chromosomal abnormality will be identified in the peripheral blood karyotype in ~12% and 5% of men, respectively. Klinefelter syndrome (47,XXY), variants of Klinefelter syndrome (e.g., 46,XY/47,XXY), or mosaicism for other chromosomal abnormalities involving aberrations in the number of X or Y chromosomes (e.g., 46,XY/45,X) account for the great majority of chromosomal abnormalities. Chromosomal rearrangements including translocations, inversions, or marker chromosomes are present in a few percent or less. Most of these men have minor or no other phenotypic abnormalities other than abnormal sperm parameters.

Deletions in *AZF* or *DAZ* gene regions of the long arm of the Y chromosome are present in about 15% of azoospermic and severely oligospermic men. The more severe the spermatogenic defect, the higher is the likelihood of a Yq microdeletion; almost all large deletions in these regions of the Y chromosome are associated with azoospermia.

Mutations in the cystic fibrosis transmembrane regulator (*CFTR*) gene are often seen in healthy men who have abnormal sperm parameters and/or non-obstructive azoospermia. Among healthy men with congenital bilateral absence of the vas deferens, about 20% are compound heterozygotes for two *CFTR* gene mutations, or compound heterozygotes for a *CFTR* mutation and a gene variant which is associated with decreased transcription of the normal gene. Another 47% carry one cystic fibrosis mutation. These data suggest that the *CFTR* gene may play a critical role in spermatogenesis or sperm physiology. Among men with abnormal sperm parameters of any kind, as many as 1 in 5 are reported to carry one cystic fibrosis mutation.

The husband should be offered peripheral blood karyotyping, chromosome Yq microdeletion testing, and cystic fibrosis mutation screening. If he carries a cystic fibrosis mutation, his wife should be offered cystic fibrosis mutation screening and/or gene sequencing.

If the husband has a chromosomal abnormality or a Yq deletion or if both members of the couple carry identifiable *CFTR* gene mutations, preimplantation genetic diagnosis could be utilized. If the husband has a chromosome Yq microdeletion each of the couple's sons would also have the microdeletion. Current information suggests that gene deletions on the Y chromosome are not medically important other than for effects on fertility.

If the husband carries a chromosomal abnormality, his siblings and other close relatives may also have the same finding. The husband should be encouraged to inform these individuals of their increased risk of fertility problems and possible risk of children with chromosomal abnormalities.

Case 3 *A 35-year-old man and his wife are referred by his urologist because an evaluation for azoospermia showed that he carries an apparently balanced chromosomal translocation: 46,XY,t(11;19)(p11.2;q13.3). His past medical history included two recent hospitalizations for pneumonia and multiple episodes of bronchitis during childhood. An episode of hemoptysis occurred a few months previously and led to a chest X-ray which revealed a right-sided heart and aortic arch with the stomach bubble located under the right hemidiaphragm. A biopsy of respiratory mucosa and examination by electron microscopy showed characteristic ultrastructural ciliary defects which are usually present in individuals affected by primary ciliary dyskinesia.*

Primary ciliary dyskinesia (PCD) is a ciliopathy, a class of genetic disorders characterized by abnormal ciliary structure and function. PCD is an autosomal recessive disorder manifested by abnormal clearance of mucus from the respiratory tract leading to chronic lung, sinus, and ear infections, which are a consequence of defective or absent cilia. About 50% of individuals with PCD also have situs inversus totalis in which there is mirror image reversal of the thoracic and abdominal organs without clinical consequences. Another 8% of affected individuals have heterotaxy in which the positions of the organs of the abdomen and chest are abnormally placed and which is associated with a high risk of congenital heart disease and other malformations. Infertility is common in males with PCD due to immotile sperm or impaired sperm motility caused by defects in the dynein arms present in the sperm tails resulting in abnormal flagellar structure.

Considerable locus heterogeneity for PCD is suspected. Mutations in two genes, *DNAH11* and *DNAH5*, are the basis for about 40% of cases. Several other genes which have not yet been identified at the time of this writing are thought to account for the remaining cases based on candidate gene analysis, positional cloning, model organism analysis, and proteomic analysis. A quantitative defect in sperm, which is present in this man, is not typical of PCD.

The man undergoes genetic testing and does not have an identifiable mutation in either his DNAH11 or DNAH5 genes, the only loci for which clinically testing is currently available.

One intriguing possibility for his azoospemia is that his chromosomal translocation disrupts a gene which is critical for normal functioning and structure of cilia. If the homolog of that gene, by chance, also has a mutation associated with PCD, this would result in disease expression. Historically, studies of individuals with an abnormal phenotype and balanced chromosomal translocations have played an important role in identifying candidate disease genes. In fact, one of the loci that has previously been implicated in PCD is at chromosome 19q13.3, which is also the site of one of the translocation breakpoints in this man. Sequencing of the breakpoints of this man's translocation might identify a nucleotide change or gene deletion that is the underlying basis for some cases of PCD. On a research basis, analysis of DNA from this man may provide important insights into the underlying molecular basis of the ciliopathies. Array comparative genomic hybridization (array CGH) would also have utility in determining whether the man's chromosomal translocation is associated with deletion or duplication which was not detected by routine metaphase analysis.

If in vitro fertilization and intracytoplasmic sperm injection result in a successful pregnancy, the couple faces an increased risk of having a child with an unbalanced chromosomal translocation. Given that the couple will need to use assisted reproductive technology to achieve a pregnancy, preimplantation genetic diagnosis for unbalanced translocations should also be considered.

The couple is concerned about the risk of a child with PCD, presuming they are able to conceive.

The risk of PCD in the couple's children depends on the carrier frequency of the gene in the general population. If the incidence of a disorder due to a specific gene is between 1 in 10 000 and 1 in 30 000, using the Hardy–Weinberg equilibrium, the disease incidence can be used to calculate a heterozygote frequency which ranges from 1 in 50 to about 1 in 90. Using 1/50 in the risk calculation, the risk of an affected child would be about 1/100 [1 (the chance that the husband carries a mutant gene) × 1/50 (the chance that the wife carries the same mutant gene) × $^1/_2$ (the chance that she transmits that gene to the child)]. This risk calculation assumes no genetic heterogeneity for PCD, an assumption that is incorrect. The actual risk for a child with PCD is much smaller because at least twelve genetic loci have been implicated in PCD. A risk of disease in the child would only exist if the wife's PCD mutation was at the same locus as her husband's. The wife's chance of being a carrier of a mutation at the same locus as her husband is smaller than the overall risk of her being a carrier of mutation in at least one locus. In the absence of an identifiable disease causing mutation in the husband or his wife, preimplantation or prenatal genetic diagnosis by molecular analysis is not possible. Ultrasonographic examination could be used to establish the fetal situs, but only half of individuals with PCD have situs inversus totalis.

Case 4   A couple is referred by their fertility specialist. Semen analysis had revealed azoospermia which prompted a chromosomal analysis for the husband. Ninety-five percent of his cells had a 46,XX karyotype and the remaining cells had a 46,XY karyotype. Testicular biopsy revealed normal-appearing testicular tissue. Sperm were noted in small quantities in one of the biopsy specimens. Physical examination of the husband revealed normal-appearing male external genitalia.

There is a wide range of effects for an individual with a mixture of XX and XY cells, ranging from normal or near normal male, to normal or near normal female, to individuals with ambiguous sexual organs. Individuals with a significant mixture of XX and XY cells have a high chance of abnormalities related to sexual development and/or sex cell development which are of variable severity. Although the husband has a high percentage of white blood cells with an XX chromosome complement, he likely has a significant percentage of cells with an XY chromosomal complement in other body tissues given his normal male appearance. The presence of the XX cell line is the most likely explanation for his impaired ability to make sperm.

Abdominal and pelvic imaging for the husband is indicated to look for evidence of any sex organ structures which would be related to having an XX cell line. If such structures were present, they may be associated with an increased risk of malignancy and endocrine and surgical consultation would be recommended.

The husband's chromosomal complement could have resulted from the early fusion of XX and XY embryos in what was originally a twin gestation, or an XXY embryo which lost an X chromosome in some cells and a Y chromosome in others to generate the XX and XY cell lines. The latter possibility could be associated with some of the husband's tissues containing some cells with a 47, XXY chromosomal complement.

The likelihood of a 47,XXY cell line being present in other tissues that we cannot easily study is unknown. If 47, XXY cells were present in the husband, this might be associated with a small increased risk of offspring with sex chromosome abnormalities (i.e., 47,XXX and 47,XXY).

There is almost no literature about the reproductive experience of individuals with the husband's chromosomal complement. Although his sperm appear normally formed, they are few in number and whether they are functionally normal and can result in successful fertilization is not known. If pregnancy is achieved via in vitro fertilization and ICSI using sperm obtained from testicular biopsy, and the pregnancy proceeds normally with normal ultrasonographic imaging, one could be reasonably optimistic about the outcome.

Further reading

1 Chodhari R, Mitchison HM, Meeks, M. (2004) Cilia, primary ciliary dyskinesia and molecular genetics. *Pediatric Respiratory Reviews* 5:69–76.

2 De Braekeleer M, Dao T-N (1990) Cytogenetic studies in couples experiencing repeated pregnancy losses. *Human Reproduction* 5:519–528.

3 Dohle GR, Halley DJ, Van Hemel JO *et al.* (2002) Genetic risk factors in infertile men with severe oligozoospermia and azoospermia. *Human Reproduction* 17 (1):13–16.

4 Hansen M, Bower C, Milne E *et al.* (2005) Assisted reproductive technologies and the risk of birth defects – a systematic review. *Human Reproduction* 20 (2):328–338.

5 Bhasin S (2007) Approach to the infertile man. *Journal of Clinical Endocrinology and Metabolism* 92(6):1995–2004.

6 Gardner RJM, Sutherland GR (2004) *Chromosome Abnormalities and Genetic Counseling*, 3rd edition. Oxford University Press.

7 Sugawara N, Tokunaga Y, Maeda M *et al.* (2005) A successful pregnancy outcome using frozen testicular sperm from a chimeric infertile male with a 46,XX/46, XY karyotype: Case report. *Human Reproduction* 20 (1):147–148.

8 Walsh TJ, Pera RR, Turek PJ (2009) The genetics of male infertility. *Seminars in Reproductive Medicine* 27 (2):124–136.

Family history

Family history of cerebral palsy

Case 1 *A woman presents for obstetric care in the first trimester. Her family history is remarkable for a brother who has cerebral palsy.*

Cerebral palsy is an umbrella term describing a constellation of clinical signs which includes spasticity, ataxia, and choreoathetotic movements due to abnormalities of the brain involved in motor function, and often mental retardation. Most cases of cerebral palsy are attributed to brain damage due to perinatal hypoxia, asphyxia, prematurity, perinatal infection, abnormal vasculature in twin gestations, hyperbilirubinemia, shaken baby syndrome, and lead poisoning. None of these causes would pose a significant risk of recurrence in our patient's own children.

Occasionally, however, the symptoms of a genetic disorder due to a single gene defect can mimic the symptoms of cerebral palsy and be misdiagnosed, as shown in Table 6.1. Misdiagnosis of a genetic disorder can have implications for other relatives who may be at high risk of having a similarly affected child. The possibility of an underlying genetic disorder may not even be considered, especially if there has been a difficult delivery when it is easy to attribute abnormal neurologic findings to presumed birth hypoxia. The neurologic abnormalities of an underlying genetic disorder may place a fetus at higher risk for a difficult delivery.

How much further investigation is necessary of a relative reported to have cerebral palsy depends on the exact relationship to the woman. Risks could be high in the setting of a previous child who has been misdiagnosed and actually has a Mendelian disorder where the recurrence risk would be 25% for a recessive disorder. Similarly, if there is an affected male relative on the maternal side (e.g., her brother, maternal uncles, or father), X-linked inheritance could pose a significant risk. Other scenarios pose less risk based on common genetic hypotheses of causation. Although a genetics evaluation of the affected individual is the ideal approach to determining whether there are risks to the patient's pregnancy, the reality is that accomplishing such evaluations is at best difficult, if it is possible at all. Usually, there is incomplete and minimal information available about the affected person with cerebral palsy, making it impossible to assess the validity of the diagnosis. When the symptoms of cerebral palsy are present, it is important to gather as much information as possible about the affected individual and the family history. In the absence of complete information, it is important to acknowledge that if the symptoms are associated with a genetic disorder, there could be a significantly increased risk of recurrence.

Upon further questioning of the woman, she reports that her 32-year-old brother was born at 29 weeks' gestation

Table 6.1 The more common disorders which may be misdiagnosed as cerebral palsy (listed alphabetically)

With apparent or real muscle weakness	*With predominant diplegia/tetraplegia*
Duchenne/Becker muscular dystrophy	Adrenoleukodystrophy, adrenomyeloneuropathy
Infantile neuroaxonal dystrophy	Arginase deficiency
Mitochondrial cytopathy	Hereditary progressive spastic paraplegia
	Holocarboxylase synthetase deficiency
With significant dystonia/involuntary movements	Metachromatic leukodystrophy
Dopa-responsive dystonia	
Glutaric aciduria type 1	*With significant ataxia*
Juvenile neuronal ceroid lipofuscinosis	Angelman syndrome
Lesch–Nyhan syndrome	Ataxia telangiectasia
Pelizaeus–Merzbacher disease	Chronic/adult GM 1 gangliosidosis
Pyruvate dehydrogenase deficiency (and other	Mitochondrial cytopathy (specifically due to the NARP mutation)
mitochondrial cytopathies presenting with	Niemann–Pick disease type C
a Leigh syndrome phenotype)	Pontocerebellar atrophy/hypoplasia (in isolation or as part
Rett syndrome	of the carbohydrate glycoprotein deficiency syndrome)
3-methylglutaconic aciduria	Posterior fossa tumor
3-methylcrotonyl CoA carboxylase deficiency	X-linked spinocerebellar ataxia

Reproduced from Gupta R, Appleton RE (2001) *Archives of Disease in Childhood* **85**(5):356–360. Reproduced with permission from BMJ Publishing Group Ltd.

and had many medical complications associated with severe prematurity during the first year of his life. The brother reportedly has mild mental retardation, dysarthria, and spasticity affecting all four extremities. His symptoms have remained unchanged over time. The woman has a large family and no other family members similarly affected.

If the brother has an X-linked recessive condition, the woman could have a significant chance of having an affected child. Had the woman's sibling been a sister, concern about an X-linked recessive condition would be much less.

How can we determine whether the patient's brother has a genetic disorder masquerading as cerebral palsy? This is usually very difficult to do, primarily because more information about the brother may not be available or may be difficult to obtain. However, there are a set of key questions which should be asked which might raise or allay suspicions.

1 Are the brother's symptoms static or progressive? The symptoms of "cerebral palsy" typically do not worsen over time. In contrast, the clinical course of some genetic disorders which are misdiagnosed as cerebral palsy may be progressive.

2 Does the brother have any unusual clinical signs? Are there abnormal eye movements? Is there self-mutilation? Are there congenital abnormalities?

3 Has the brother had brain imaging or an evaluation by a geneticist?

4 Is there a family history of other similarly affected individuals? Some genetic disorders may have more or less severe manifestations in other family members.

The history of significant prematurity, especially 32 years ago, and the lack of progression of symptoms provides reasonable reassurance in this scenario that a brain insult in the perinatal period is the most probable explanation for the brother's problems. However, if this brother is available, the family can be offered a genetics evaluation on this individual.

Case 2 A woman reports that her 30-year-old brother was born at term after a difficult delivery. He has severe spasticity of his lower extremities, mild spasticity of his upper extremities, and is largely wheelchair bound. The diagnosis of "cerebral palsy" due to presumptive birth hypoxia after a difficult delivery was made after an evaluation at age 6 years. He has normal intelligence, is a college graduate, and is living independently. He has had

abnormal eye movements noted since infancy which have not impaired his vision. Upon further questioning, the woman reports that her 14-month-old son has delayed motor milestones and identical eye movements to those seen in her brother.

Cerebral palsy is often associated with normal intelligence so this aspect of the brother's history does not provide any useful clues. Abnormal eye movements are not typical of cerebral palsy and warrant further investigation. Given that the woman's son also has abnormal eye movements, we now have a significant concern about an underlying familial genetic condition. Genetics evaluations of the brother and son are recommended.

The son was hypotonic and ataxic. Ophthalmologic evaluation revealed horizontal nystagmus for both individuals. Magnetic resonance imaging of the brother revealed white matter disease. The clinical findings were consistent with Pelizaeus–Merzbacher disease, a rare X-linked dysmyelinating disorder which has a highly variable clinical presentation in both males and females and which is caused by mutations in the *PLP1* gene. Gene sequencing of the *PLP1* genes of the patient's son and brother identified a disease-causing mutation, thereby allowing for prenatal genetic diagnosis in this pregnancy and preimplantation genetic diagnosis in future pregnancies.

Case 3 A woman reports that her 26-year-old brother was noted to have delayed motor milestones by 8 months of age. He never walked and is wheelchair bound. He is described as having cerebral palsy with choreoathetotic movements beginning around age 3 years. He has mild mental retardation. He has had recurrent problems with kidney stones and recently developed arthritis in his great toes. No other family members are similarly affected.

The presence of kidney stones and signs of gouty arthritis in a young man are unusual and should raise consideration of a disorder associated with uric acid overproduction. Lesch–Nyhan disease is an X-linked disorder associated with hyperuricemia due to deficiency of the enzyme hypoxanthine-guanine phosphoribosyltransferase (HPRT). In the classic form, self-injurious behavior including biting of the hands, fingers, and lips leads to severe mutilation. However, as for most genetic diseases, there is a wide clinical spectrum and not all affected individuals have self-mutilating behavior. In the above scenario, the presence of unusual medical problems not typical of cerebral palsy raises concerns about an underlying genetic disorder. A genetics evaluation of the brother is indicated.

The brother's evaluation reveals hyperuricemia and HPRT enzyme activity less than 2% of normal. A mutation was identified in his *HPRT1* gene. His sister, our patient, was subsequently identified as heterozygous for the mutation. Prenatal genetic diagnosis can be performed in the current pregnancy and preimplantation diagnosis is possible in future pregnancies.

Further reading

1 Fattal-Valevski A, DiMaio MS, Hisama FM *et al.* (2009) Variable expression of a novel PLP1 mutation in members of a family with Pelizaeus-Merzbacher disease. *Journal of Child Neurology* **24**:618–624.

2 Gupta R, Appleton RE (2001) Cerebral palsy: not always what it seems. *Archives of Diseases in Childhood* **85**;356–360.

Family history of non-specific mental retardation

Case 1 A primiparous woman who has a postgraduate degree is referred for genetic counseling because a deceased maternal uncle had mental retardation. He was moderately retarded without any unusual facial features or other physical findings. No medical records are available for review. Her karyotype is normal.

Mental retardation is etiologically heterogeneous with genetic and environmental causes. A large number of genetic syndromes with Mendelian inheritance are associated with cognitive deficits of variable severity. Without more information about the underlying cause of the uncle's mental retardation and the patient's family history, it is not possible to provide accurate information about the risk of recurrence in her family.

A detailed family history should be collected when mental retardation is present in a close relative. The presence of other relatives, who may be more mildly or severely affected than the affected uncle, and causes of death for all first- and second-degree relatives should be ascertained. Specific queries should be made about stillbirths and miscarriages which may not be spontaneously reported.

The number of male relatives and their relationship to the patient can sometimes be used to help increase or decrease the likelihood of X-linked inheritance.

The patient reports another maternal uncle with normal intelligence. Both maternal grandparents lived into their 70s and died of diabetes-related complications. The woman has two younger sisters. She has a small extended family. Photographs of the uncle provided by the family reveal a non-dysmorphic facies. Consanguinity is denied.

No further information about the uncle or the family history will be forthcoming. By report he did not have a degenerative condition nor did he have major malformations, thereby narrowing the diagnostic possibilities. Although the mentally retarded uncle could have had one of many Mendelian disorders, only those with X-linked inheritance pose a significant risk to the patient's children.

The most common genetic cause of mental retardation in males and females after Down syndrome is fragile X syndrome. Fragile X syndrome is a CGG trinucleotide repeat expansion disorder caused by mutations in the *FMR1* gene on the X chromosome. All males with full mutations (>200 CGG repeats) and about half of females will have cognitive impairment of variable severity. Premutations are unstable when transmitted from women and prone to expansion to full mutations with the risk of expansion correlated with the size of the premutation. Premutations in males are stable when transmitted. However, male premutation carriers have a significant risk for developing fragile X tremor and ataxia syndrome (FXTAS) in mid to later life. The risk of FXTAS appears to be small in female premutation carriers, but these women have a 20% risk of experiencing premature ovarian failure.

Testing for the *FMR1* gene expansion is widely available and fragile X syndrome carrier testing is offered to all pregnant women at many medical centers. In the setting of a relative with mental retardation and/or autistic spectrum disorder of unknown cause, fragile X syndrome carrier testing should be offered to the patient.

If the woman's fragile X syndrome study is normal (i.e., she has normal-sized *FMR1* genes), there is currently no further testing that could practically be offered to look for other causes of X-linked mental retardation. Although there are at least 15 genes known to be associated with non-syndromic X-linked mental retardation (i.e., mental retardation unassociated with birth defects and dysmorphology), and many more suspected, it is not yet practical to analyze these genes unless an affected family member has a documented mutation.

Case 2 A woman and her husband are referred for genetic counseling because first trimester screening predicted an increased risk for Down syndrome. Upon collecting the couple's histories, you learn that both of them have severe learning disabilities and attended special schools; they live independently and deny any health problems. Their parents and siblings all have college degrees. The couple is concerned about having a child with learning disabilities.

Learning disabilities and borderline mental retardation can be familial and reflect the lower spectrum of the normal IQ distribution. This explanation seems unlikely for this couple because of the high educational achievements of their parents and siblings. Alternatively, low normal or borderline IQ may represent a discrete genetic abnormality.

Further testing of this couple to investigate the cause of their learning difficulties could include:
- standard metaphase chromosomal analysis to look for gross chromosomal abnormalities;
- fragile X syndrome carrier testing for the woman;
- formal genetics evaluation to look for subtle dysmorphic features that could lead to a more focused investigation;
- array comparative genomic hybridization (array CGH).

These tests have only a small chance of identifying the cause of the couple's learning difficulties. In most situations, the problems go unexplained.

The woman has a normal peripheral blood karyotype, and array CGH study, and a negative fragile X study. Her husband has two small alterations on the short arm of chromosome 6 by array CGH. One is a small deletion (2 Mb) and adjacent to it is a small duplication (0.8 Mb).

Array CGH is a molecular cytogenetic method which is more sensitive than standard metaphase karyotyping in detecting chromosomal imbalances. One adverse consequence of array CGH is the recognition of gene copy number variants that are of unknown clinical significance. In this case, we recommend that the husband's parents have chromosomal analysis with array CGH. If the deletion/duplication is inherited from a parent who does not have any phenotypic abnormalities, it is more likely to represent a normal chromosomal variant in this family. On the other hand, if the deletion/duplication has arisen de novo in the husband, it is more likely, but not certain, that it is associated with the learning difficulties noted in the husband.

The husband's parents have normal peripheral blood karyotypes and array CGH studies (neither has the duplication/deletion of the short arm of chromosome 6). The woman elects to undergo amniocentesis due to the increased risk for Down syndrome predicted by first trimester screening. The amniocyte karyotype is 46,XY; array CGH shows that the fetus inherited his father's deletion/duplication on chromosome 6.

Predictions about the effects on the fetus of the deletion/duplication on chromosome 6p are difficult to make. There are no case reports in the literature of a similar chromosomal finding. We presume that the husband's chromosomal abnormality is an important etiologic factor for his learning difficulties although that conclusion cannot be made with certainty. If our presumption is correct, the fetus will most likely have learning problems which are at a minimum similar to those of the husband. There is a potential for more severe effects on cognitive functioning because the wife also has learning difficulties which could have an unidentified genetic component. In addition, the expression of genes of interest on chromosome 6 in the fetus will be influenced by the wife's genotype on chromosome 6p and elsewhere. There could also be subtle changes in the deletion/duplication during transmission to the fetus.

Consanguinity

Case 1 A 36-year-old Indian woman and her husband are referred for genetic counseling because of advanced maternal age. The woman's family history includes her brother's daughter who is reported to have spina bifida. The woman and her husband are first cousins. The woman's mother is the sister of the husband's father.

The offspring of first cousin marriages have a risk of birth defects and mental retardation which is 5–6% or about double that of offspring of unrelated parents. This risk is due to the increased likelihood of homozygosity for recessive mutant genes and for mutations associated with polygenic or multifactorial disorders. First cousins share 1/8 or 12.5% of their genes which are inherited from their common grandparents. Therefore, for any allele carried by one member of this couple there is a 1/8 chance that the partner has inherited the same allele from a common ancestral source. If one partner passes this allele to the offspring there is 1/16 (1/8 × $^1/_2$) or 6.25% chance that both alleles in the offspring of a first cousin mating will be identical by descent. Repeated generations of consanguineous matings are associated with a significantly increased risk for rare single gene disorders because a greater fraction of genes will be from common ancestors. Matings between individuals who have a second cousin or more remote relationship do not have an increased risk of birth defects and classic genetic disorders over the general population risk of about 3% if the family history does not include relatives who have a known autosomal recessive condition.

In this couple's situation, the risk for having a child with a neural tube defect, a multifactorial disorder, is increased because the relative with spina bifida is both the woman's niece and the husband's first cousin once removed. This increases the probability of genetic loading in the couple's offspring for susceptibility genes conferring an increased risk of neural tube defects.

There is no specific testing that can be offered to consanguineous couples unless there are known autosomal recessive disorders in the family other than routine screening for disorders that have a high frequency among individuals of their ancestral background or geographic origin. In this couple's situation, their Indian ancestry places both of them at increased risk for carrying hemoglobin variants which in the homozygous form would lead to a serious inherited anemia (e.g., beta thalassemia, hemoglobin E/beta thalassemia, sickle cell disorders) and for which both prenatal and preimplantation genetic diagnosis is available. If one member of the couple carries a hemoglobin variant, the chance that the other member of the couple also carries this hemoglobin variant is 1/8, which is increased over the population carrier frequency.

Folic acid supplementation beginning prior to conception and continuing throughout the first trimester would also be recommended for the woman to decrease the risk of occurrence of a neural tube defect. Fetal ultrasonography is the most sensitive test to diagnose this condition.

Case 2 A couple seeks genetic counseling regarding the risk of recurrence in a future pregnancy of the abnormalities present in their 10-year-old son who has mental retardation, short stature, renal disease requiring dialysis diagnosed at age 4 years, minor facial dysmorphology including dental crowding, down-slanting palpebral fissures, and posteriorly rotated ears. An extensive genetics evaluation including routine chromosomal analysis, metabolic evaluation, and chromosomal array CGH did not identify an underlying cause for his problems. He was normal-appearing at birth. The examining geneticist felt that the son's abnormalities may well represent a novel single gene disorder. The couple also has two normally developing daughters. The couple are third cousins; the wife's great grandmother was the sister of the husband's great grandmother. No other family members are known to have problems similar to that of the son.

In the absence of an underlying genetic diagnosis, providing an accurate risk of recurrence of the son's problems and prenatal diagnosis is not possible. If the disorder is X-linked or autosomal recessive, the risk of recurrence would be 25%. Autosomal recessive inheritance might be favored here given the parents' consanguinity, but the couple only shares 1/128 of their genes. However, an X-linked disorder remains a possibility, although mutant genes on the X chromosome and their phenotypes have been extensively described and none match the description of the son's abnormalities. If his disorder were due to a new dominant mutation, the risk of recurrence would be small, but slightly increased over the background risk due to the small chance of gonadal mosaicism for the mutation in one of the parents. Unfortunately, there is no testing of the parents or of the pregnancy that can provide definitive information for them.

Further reading

1 Bennett RL, Motulsky AG, Bittles A *et al.* (2002) Genetic Counseling and Screening of Consanguineous Couples and Their Offspring: Recommendations of the National Society of Genetic Counselors. *Journal of Genetic Counseling* **11**:97–119.

2 Bittles AH (2001) Consanguinity and its relevance to clinical practice. *Clinical Genetics* **60**:89–98.

Non-paternity

Case 1 *A 32-year-old woman is referred for consultation by her obstetrician because she and her husband have a 2-year-old daughter affected with Niemann–Pick disease type C (NPC), an autosomal recessive neurodegenerative disorder caused by inability to degrade cholesterol resulting in accumulation of cholesterol and other fats in multiple organs including the brain. The most severe form of the disorder is associated with a neurodegenerative course in early childhood. Review of the daughter's medical record confirms the diagnosis of NPC; analysis of her cultured fibroblasts showed impaired cholesterol esterification and positive filipin staining, the best biochemical tests for diagnosing this disorder at the time. Filipin staining refers to a characteristic fluorescence pattern in the nucleus of fibroblasts which have abnormal accumulation of unes-terified cholesterol.*

Risk of recurrence of NPC is 25%. Biochemical testing of chorionic villus cells or amniocytes to demonstrate impaired cholesterol esterification is not available. If the disease-causing mutations are documented in the family, definitive prenatal or preimplantation genetic diagnosis would be available for future pregnancies. NPC is genetically heterogeneous. This refers to the situation where mutations in different underlying genes can result in the same clinical phenotype. Two *NPC* genes have been identified; about 95% of affected individuals have mutations in the *NPC1* gene and the remaining individuals have mutations in the *NPC2* gene. Molecular testing can find the majority of disease-causing mutations. Blood samples for DNA extraction are collected from the affected daughter and both parents. Identification of the disease-causing mutations in the parents will allow carrier detection for the parents' siblings and other interested relatives.

The results of molecular analysis indicate that the affected daughter has two previously characterized pathogenic mutations in her NPC1 genes. She is a compound hetero-zygote for a frameshift mutation leading to a stop codon and for a partial gene deletion. Analysis of the parents' DNA samples indicates that the mother carries the mis-sense mutation; the father does not carry the partial gene deletion; sequencing of his NPC1 gene does not identify any sequence variants.

Analysis of the father's peripheral blood DNA does not show evidence of the *NPC1* gene mutation which is present in his daughter.

Non-paternity is the most likely explanation for the results of molecular analysis. Non-paternity rates vary widely among populations; in North America, estimates suggest a rate of 5% or higher.

Another explanation is a sample error which resulted in analysis of another person's DNA. A sample error could occur at the time of phlebotomy or in the laboratory. Large studies of sample identification errors in clinical laboratory testing indicate that the frequency of misla-beled samples ranges widely among different laboratories and in different areas of the world.

A new mutation in the father's sperm is another possibility. The new mutation rate for autosomal recessive genes varies widely and ranges from 1 in a million to about 1%. De novo *NPC1* gene mutations are considered rare.

The mother should be informed of these explanations in a private consultation without other family members present. If non-paternity is not acknowledged, another blood sample from her husband to address the possibility of sample error is indicated. Because of the possibility that the father has gonadal mosaicism for the partial *NPC1* gene deletion, prenatal diagnosis for the disease-causing mutations should be offered in future pregnancies.

The molecular genetics laboratory could also do paternity testing on the original DNA samples it received. Confirmation that the father and daughter are related would eliminate the possibility of sample error and provide strong evidence for a de novo mutation occurring in the father's sperm. If the father's and daughter's DNA samples are not compatible, both non-paternity and a sample error would remain possibilities.

Whether paternity is established or not, prenatal diagnosis could be elected in future pregnancies with testing for the two mutations present in the couple's daughter.

Further reading

1 College of American Pathologists, Valenstein PN, Raab SS *et al.* (2006) Identification errors involving clinical laboratories: a College of American Pathologists Q-Probes study of patient and specimen identification errors at 120 institutions. *Archives of Pathology and Laboratory Medicine* **130**:1106–1113.

2 Dzik WH, Murphy MF, Andreu G *et al.* (2003) An international study of the performance of sample collection from patients. *Vox Sanguinis* **85**:40–47.

3 Lucassen A, Parker M (2001) Revealing false paternity: some ethical considerations. *Lancet* **357**:1033–1035.

4 Vanier MT, Millat G (2003) Niemann–Pick disease type C. *Clinical Genetics* **64**:269–281.

Fetal infection

Case 1 *A 24-year-old woman is referred for detailed ultrasonographic examination at 17 weeks' gestation because biochemical serum screening predicted a 1 in 40 risk for Down syndrome. Ultrasonographic examination reveals two intracranial lesions, which are suspected to be calcifications, and mild fetal hydrops.*

Intracranial calcifications with or without fetal hydrops are strongly suggestive of an infectious cause such as toxoplasmosis, cytomegalovirus, herpes simplex virus or varicella. Intracranial calcifications are seen rarely in the setting of an inherited disorder.

Serologic testing of the mother is ordered to look for evidence of parvovirus B19 and TORCH infections (toxoplasma, rubella, cytomegalovirus, herpes simplex virus), and an amniocentesis is performed. The fetal karyotype is normal. The results of serologic tests reveal positive toxoplasma IgG and IgM. Serology for parvovirus B19, rubella, cytomegalovirus, and herpes simplex virus shows evidence of past infections. The woman reports no medical problems during the pregnancy. She has cats at home and changes a litter box. She gardens without gloves.

Primary toxoplasmosis infections are usually asymptomatic in a pregnant woman. The patient has serologic evidence of a toxoplasmosis infection and has associated risk factors. Whether the woman has had a recent toxoplasmosis infection or one in the distant past cannot be determined from the results of her serology. IgM antibodies appear early in acute toxoplasmosis infection but

can persist for longer than a year. Besides intracranial calcifications, other features of toxoplasmosis embryopathy that may be evident in utero in the second trimester include hydrocephalus, cataracts, microcephaly, hepatosplenomegaly, hydrops, and intrauterine growth restriction. For cases such as this woman's where routine serology cannot distinguish between an acute or previously acquired infection, an algorithm for further and more complex serologic testing at a specialized laboratory such as the Palo Alto Medical Foundation Toxoplasma Serology Laboratory is recommended. Establishing the timing of the infection will influence decisions about whether to initiate maternal drug treatment and pursue diagnostic testing of the fetus.

The risk of congenital infection is dependent on gestational age at the time of seroconversion with risks of about 6%, 40%, and 72%, depending on whether seroconversion occurs in the first, second, or third trimester, respectively. However, among fetuses with congenital infection, the probability of developing clinical features of toxoplasmosis embryopathy and the severity of those features before age 3 years is inversely correlated with gestational age at the time of maternal seroconversion with risks of 60%, 25%, and 9% for maternal infections acquired in the first, second, or third trimesters, respectively.

Invasive testing by amniocentesis to test for the toxoplasma organism in amniotic fluid by polymerase chain reaction is recommended when maternal serology suggests a recently acquired infection and when fetal ultrasonographic examination reveals abnormalities suggestive of or consistent with toxoplasmosis embryopathy. Decisions regarding invasive testing for immunosuppressed women who are at risk for reactivation of a latent

Prenatal Diagnosis: Cases & Clinical Challenges, 1st edition.   By Miriam S. DiMaio, Joyce E. Fox, Maurice J. Mahoney
Published 2010 by Blackwell Publishing Ltd.

toxoplasmosis infection must take into account the underlying maternal disease state as HIV infection may be a contraindication to amniocentesis.

The results of maternal serology performed in a reference laboratory confirms the evidence for an acute toxoplasmosis infection in the mother. Polymerase chain reaction testing of amniotic fluid is positive for toxoplasma DNA, confirming a fetal infection. The woman is informed that the fetus has a significant chance of suffering from complications of a congenital toxoplasmosis infection. The woman plans to continue the pregnancy.

Treatment with antibiotics has been shown to be effective in reducing the probability of maternal to fetal transmission and in reducing the severity of abnormalities in affected fetuses. In general, recommendations for treatment of women in whom toxoplasmosis is confirmed or suspected to have been acquired during the pregnancy will be influenced by the gestational age at which the maternal infection was acquired and the results of molecular testing for toxoplasma DNA in amniotic fluid. Because maternal treatment can be associated with both maternal and fetal toxicity, experts in the management of acute toxoplasmosis infections should be consulted. In the United States, two sources are the Palo Alto Medical Foundation Toxoplasma Serology Laboratory and the US National Collaborative Treatment Trial Study in Chicago.

Further reading

1 Montoya JG, Remington JS (2008) Management of Toxoplasma gondii infection during pregnancy. *Clinical Infectious Diseases* **47**:554–66.

Teratogens

A 28-year-old Caucasian woman is referred for genetic counseling in her first pregnancy after the sonographic diagnosis of a fetal meningomyelocele at 18 weeks' gestation. No other fetal defects are apparent and the fetal karyotype is normal. She has been treated for several years and throughout the pregnancy with valproic acid for an idiopathic seizure disorder which began in her teens. She remained seizure-free during the pregnancy. Her family history includes a sister who also has a seizure disorder treated with valproic acid and who has four healthy children each of whom was exposed to valproic acid in utero. No relative of the woman or her husband has a neural tube defect.

In utero exposure to valproic acid is associated with an increased risk of congenital malformations, craniofacial dysmorphology, and neurodevelopmental abnormalities. Fetal exposure during organogenesis is associated with a 1 to 2% risk of neural tube defects, mainly lumbosacral meningomyelocele. There is also an increased risk of other malformations, primarily heart and radial limb reduction defects and hypospadias. Published studies show that the overall risk for major malformations among the offspring of mothers treated with valproic acid ranges from 6% to 18%. The risk of abnormalities is highest among women being treated with high doses of valproic acid and those who are being treated with valproic acid and one or more other anticonvulsants.

There is also an increased risk of facial dysmorphology, which is shared with several other anticonvulsants. Findings include a long and thin upper lip, a shallow philtrum, epicanthal folds, and midface hypoplasia manifested by a flat nasal bridge, small upturned nose, and downturned angles of the mouth. Intrauterine growth restriction may also be present. The magnitude of this risk is not well established.

A significant risk of decreased intellectual capacity, neurodevelopmental abnormalities, and autistic spectrum disorder is reported in children who were exposed in utero to valproic acid. However, studies which have evaluated the magnitude of the risk of this component of valproic acid embryopathy are limited by multiple confounding factors including socioeconomic status, maternal drug and alcohol use, cigarette smoking, and maternal seizures during pregnancy.

Most recent studies show that maternal epilepsy, when well controlled during the pregnancy, does not significantly increase the risk of birth defects.

The woman wants to understand why her sister's children have not suffered adverse effects from their in utero valproic acid exposure.

The underlying cause of non-syndromic neural tube defects is presumed to be the combined interactions of genetic and environmental susceptibility factors. Even for a woman treated with anticonvulsants who has had one child with a neural tube defect, the risk for recurrence of a second affected child, while increased to several percent, is not 100%. The lack of concordance for the abnormal phenotype in subsequent children even with the same intrauterine exposure to valproic acid reflects, in part, the different genetic backgrounds of siblings who share, on average, only 50% of their genes.

Murine models suggest that about 200 genes with diverse functions are involved in the genesis of neural tube defects. In addition, there is an additional contribution to the etiology of neural tube defects that may be attributable to postzygotic genetic changes, epigenetic phenomena, and effects of the placental vascular supply as suggested by twin studies which show that not all monozygotic twins have concordance for a neural tube defect.

> *In anticipation of another pregnancy, the woman consults with her neurologist who reports that valproic acid is the only anticonvulsant that has effectively controlled this woman's seizures.*

Women who require anticonvulsant therapy should be treated because uncontrolled seizures pose a higher risk to the fetus and the woman compared with the teratogenic risks. Valproic acid has high teratogenicity; alternative anticonvulsant medications should be used if at all possible. Unfortunately, for this woman, valproic acid appears to be her only choice.

Folic acid has been shown to reduce the recurrence of neural tube defects, heart defects, and facial clefting. Valproic acid is an antimetabolite to folic acid, while other commonly used anticonvulsants interfere with intestinal absorption of folic acid. There are conflicting data about whether folic acid supplementation is effective in reducing the risk of valproic acid-related neural tube defects.

Murine models show that protective effects of folate supplementation vary among different genetic strains of mice that harbor different susceptibility mutations for neural tube defects. The limited experience with human pregnancies has thus far not demonstrated effectiveness of folic acid in reducing the risk of valproic acid embryopathy in exposed fetuses. Nonetheless, it is recommended that women being treated with valproic acid during pregnancy be treated with 4 mg/day of folic acid beginning one month prior to conception and continuing through the first trimester of pregnancy.

Further reading

1 Fried S, Kozer E, Nulman I *et al.* (2004) Malformation rates in children of women with untreated epilepsy. *Drug Safety* **27**:197–202.

2 Genton P, Semach F, Trinka E (2006) Valproic acid in epilepsy: pregnancy related issues. *Drug Safety* **29**:1–21.

3 Hall JG (1996) Twinning: mechanisms and genetic implications. *Current Opinion in Genetics and Development* **6**:343–347.

4 Harris MJ (2009) Insights into prevention of human neural tube defects by folic acid arising from consideration of mouse mutants. *Birth Defects Research A: Clinical Molecular Teratology* **85**:331–339.

5 Kaaja E, Kaaja R, Hiilesmaa V (2003) Major malformations in offspring of women with epilepsy. *Neurology* **60** (4):575–579.

6 Ornoy A (2009) Valproic acid in pregnancy: How much are we endangering the embryo and fetus. *Reproductive Toxicology* **28**:1–10.

7 Yerby MS (2003) Management issues for women with epilepsy: neural tube defects and folic acid supplementation. *Neurology* **61**:S23–26.

Appendix

Acrocentric chromosome: A chromosome that has its centromere near the end. The human acrocentric chromosomes are 13, 14, 15, 21, and 22.

Allele:[*] One of the alternative versions of a gene at a given location (locus) along a chromosome.

Array comparative genomic hybridization (array CGH):[**] A technique that allows the detection of losses and gains in DNA copy number across the entire genome without prior knowledge of specific chromosomal abnormalities. Array CGH is also called chromosome microarray.

Aneuploidy:[*] The occurrence of one or more extra or missing chromosomes leading to an unbalanced chromosome complement; or any chromosome number that is not an exact multiple of the haploid number.

Anticipation:[*] The tendency in certain genetic disorders for individuals in successive generations to present at an earlier age and/or with more severe manifestations; often observed in disorders resulting from the expression of a trinucleotide repeat mutation that tends to increase in size and have a more significant effect when passed from one generation to the next.

Autosome:[***] Any chromosome other than a sex chromosome. Humans have 22 pairs of autosomes.

Bayes' theorem: A mathematical calculation of probability that incorporates incidents that have already occurred to revise the probability of a given event.

Chromosomal inversion:[*] A chromosomal rearrangement in which a segment of genetic material is broken away from the chromosome, inverted from end to end, and reinserted into the chromosome at the same breakage site. Balanced inversions (no net loss or gain of genetic material) are usually not associated with phenotypic abnormalities, although in some cases gene disruptions at the breakpoints can cause adverse phenotypic effects, including some known genetic diseases; unbalanced inversions (loss or gain of chromosome material) usually yield an abnormal phenotype.

Chromosomal rearrangement:[*] A structural alteration in a chromosome, usually involving breakage and reattachment of a segment of chromosome material, resulting in an abnormal configuration; examples include inversions and translocations.

Chromosomal translocation:[*] A chromosome alteration in which a whole chromosome or segment of a chromosome becomes attached to or interchanged with another whole chromosome or segment, the resulting hybrid segregating together at meiosis; balanced translocations (in which there is no net loss or gain of chromosome material) are usually not associated with phenotypic abnormalities, although gene disruptions at the breakpoints of the translocation can, in some cases, cause adverse effects, including some known genetic disorders; unbalanced translocations (in which there is loss or gain of chromosome material) usually yield an abnormal phenotype.

Cis configuration:[*] Term which indicates that an individual who is heterozygous at two neighboring loci has the two mutations in question on the same chromosome.

Clastogen: A substance that causes chromosomal breakage.

Compound heterozygote:[*] An individual who has two different abnormal alleles at a particular locus, one on each chromosome of a pair; usually refers to individuals affected with an autosomal recessive disorder.

Consanguinity[*]: Genetic relatedness between individuals descended from at least one common ancestor.

Deletion: A mutation in which part of a chromosome or sequence of DNA is missing.

De novo mutation:[*] An alteration in a gene that is present for the first time in one family member as a result of a

---

Prenatal Diagnosis: Cases & Clinical Challenges, 1st edition. By Miriam S. DiMaio, Joyce E. Fox, Maurice J. Mahoney
Published 2010 by Blackwell Publishing Ltd.

mutation in a germ cell (egg or sperm) of one of the parents or in the fertilized egg itself.

Diploid:* The normal number of chromosomes in a somatic cell; in humans, 46 chromosomes (22 pairs of autosomes and two sex chromosomes).

Dominant negative mutation:* A mutation whose gene product adversely affects the normal, wild-type gene product within the same cell, often by dimerizing (combining) with it. In cases of polymeric molecules, such as collagen, dominant negative mutations are often more deleterious than mutations causing the production of no gene product (null mutations or null alleles).

Duplication: A mutation in which part of a chromosome or sequence of DNA is duplicated, resulting in extra genetic material.

Epigenetic:** Changes in the regulation of the expression of gene activity without alteration of genetic structure.

Fluorescence in situ hybridization (FISH):# A physical mapping approach that uses fluorescent tags to detect hybridization of probes with metaphase chromosomes and with the less-condensed somatic interphase chromatin.

Founder effect:* A gene mutation observed in high frequency in a specific population due to the presence of that gene mutation in a single ancestor or small number of ancestors.

Gamete:** Also known as sex cells or germ cells, they are the cells that come together during fertilization or conception in organisms that reproduce sexually. Their genetic complement consists of a single set of unpaired chromosomes.

Gamete compensation: Mitotic duplication of a chromosome in a cell that was monosomic for that chromosome, resulting in restoration of the diploid number with uniparental disomy for that chromosome.

Gamete complementation: The fusion of a gamete which is nullisomic for a specific chromosome with a gamete that is disomic for that chromosome, resulting in the normal diploid chromosomal complement with uniparental disomy for that chromosome.

Genetic load: The proportion of deleterious genes in an individual or in a population.

Genetic or locus heterogeneity: A disorder or trait that can result from mutations in more than one gene.

Genome:*** All the DNA contained in an organism or a cell, which includes both the chromosomes within the nucleus and the DNA in mitochondria.

Genomic imprinting:* The process by which maternally and paternally derived chromosomes are uniquely chemically modified leading to different expression of a certain gene or genes on those chromosomes depending on their parental origin.

Genotype:* The genetic constitution of an organism or cell; also refers to the specific set of alleles inherited at a locus.

Germline:* The cell line from which egg or sperm cells (gametes) are derived.

Germline mosaicism:* Two or more genetic or cytogenetic cell lines confined to the precursor (germline) cells of the egg or sperm; also called gonadal mosaicism.

Haploid:* Half the diploid or normal number of chromosomes in a somatic cell; the number of chromosomes in a gamete (egg or sperm) cell, which in humans is 23 chromosomes, one chromosome from each chromosome pair.

Hemizygous:* Describes an individual who has only one member of a chromosome pair or chromosome segment rather than the usual two; refers in particular to X-linked genes in males who under usual circumstances have only one X chromosome.

Heteroplasmy:* The situation in which, within a single cell, there is a mixture of mitochondria (energy-producing cytoplasmic organelles), some containing mutant DNA and some containing normal DNA.

Heterotaxy: Abnormal positioning of organs because of failure to establish the normal left-right pattern in the embryo; often associated with congenital heart disease, polysplenia, or asplenia.

Heterozygous:** Having two different allelic forms of a gene, one inherited from each parent, on each of the two homologous chromosomes.

Homologous chromosomes:* The two chromosomes from a particular pair, normally one inherited from the mother and one from the father, containing the same genetic loci in the same order.

Homozygous:*** Possessing two identical forms of a particular gene, one inherited from each parent.

Imprinting:* The process by which maternally and paternally derived chromosomes are uniquely chemically modified leading to different expression of a certain gene or genes on those chromosomes depending on their parental origin.

Interfamilial variability:* Variability in clinical presentation of a particular disorder among affected individuals from different families.

Interstitial deletion: A deletion that does not involve the terminal end of a chromosome.

Intracytoplasmic sperm injection (ICSI): An assisted reproductive technique in which a sperm is injected directly into the cytoplasm of an egg.

Intrafamilial variability:* Variability in clinical presentation of a particular disorder among affected individuals within the same immediate or extended family.

In vitro fertilization (IVF): The process which involves the fertilization of ovum with sperm outside of the womb in a laboratory.

Linkage analysis:* Testing DNA sequence polymorphisms (normal variants) that are near or within a gene of interest to track within a family the inheritance of a disease-causing mutation in a given gene.

Lyonization:* The phenomenon by which one X chromosome in females (either maternally derived or paternally derived) is randomly inactivated in early embryonic cells, with fixed inactivation in all descendant cells.

Metaphase karyotype: A representation of all the metaphase chromosomes within a cell.

Meiosis:** A specialized cell division in which a single diploid cell undergoes two nuclear divisions following a single round of DNA replication in order to produce four daughter cells that contain half the number of chromosomes as the diploid cell. Meiosis occurs during the formation of gametes from diploid organisms.

Methylation:* Attachment of methyl groups to DNA cytosine bases; genes that are methylated are not expressed; methylation plays a role in X-chromosome inactivation and imprinting.

Mitochondria:* Cytoplasmic organelles that produce the energy source ATP for most chemical reactions in the body and contain their own distinct genome. Mutations in mitochondrial genes are responsible for several recognized syndromes and are always maternally inherited since ova contain mitochondria, whereas sperm do not.

Mitosis:# The process of nuclear division in cells that produces daughter cells that are genetically identical to each other and to the parent cell.

Monosomy:* The presence of only one chromosome from a pair; partial monosomy refers to the presence of only one copy of a segment of a chromosome.

Mosaicism: The presence of two or more cell populations in one individual that differ in genetic make-up, either in chromosomes or in genes. The term is also applied to cells in vitro that have come from one individual.

Multifactorial inheritance:* The combined contribution of one or more often unspecified genetic and environmental factors, often, unknown, in the causation of a particular trait or disease.

Mutagen: A substance that causes changes in the DNA

Mutation:* Any alteration in a gene from its natural state; may be disease-causing or a benign, normal variant.

Non-disjunction: Failure of separation of homologous chromosomes during meiosis or mitosis.

Non-homologous chromosomes: Chromosomes that do not pair with each other during meiosis and do not have similar DNA sequences.

Omphalocele:** A congenital defect with major fissure in the abdominal wall at the umbilicus resulting in the extrusion of viscera through the umbilicus. Unlike gastroschisis, omphalocele is covered with peritoneum but without overlying skin.

PCR:* Polymerase chain reaction; A procedure that produces millions of copies of a short segment of DNA through repeated cycles of: (1) denaturation, (2) annealing, and (3) elongation; PCR is a very common procedure in molecular genetic testing and may be used to generate a sufficient quantity of DNA to perform a test.

PGD: See preimplantation genetic diagnosis.

Penetrance:* The proportion of individuals with a mutation causing a particular disorder who exhibit clinical symptoms of that disorder; a condition (most commonly inherited in an autosomal dominant manner) is said to have complete penetrance if clinical symptoms are present in all individuals who have the disease-causing mutation, and to have reduced or incomplete penetrance if clinical symptoms are not always present in individuals who have the disease-causing mutation.

Phenocopy: Similar or identical observable characteristics or abnormalities which have a different underlying genetic basis.

Phenotype:* The observable physical and/or biochemical characteristics of the expression of a gene; the clinical presentation of an individual with a particular genotype.

Polygenic:* A condition caused by the additive contributions of mutations in multiple genes at different loci.

Polymerase chain reaction: See PCR.

Polymorphism:* Natural variations in a gene, DNA sequence, protein, or chromosome that usually have no adverse effect on the individual and occur with fairly high frequency in the general population; the fairly high frequency is sometimes defined as 1% or greater.

Population risk:* The proportion of individuals in the general population who are affected with a particular disorder or who carry a certain gene; often discussed in the genetic counseling process as a comparison to the patient's personal risk given his or her family history, laboratory test results, or other circumstances.

Postzygotic event:* A mutational event or abnormality in chromosome replication/segregation that occurs after fertilization of the ovum by the sperm, often leading to mosaicism (two or mre genetically distinct cell lines within the same organism).

Preimplantation genetic diagnosis (PGD):* A procedure used to decrease the chance of a particular genetic condition for which the fetus is specifically at risk by testing one or more cells removed from early embryos conceived by in vitro fertilization and transferring to the mother's uterus only those embryos determined not to have inherited the mutation in question.

Pseudoautosomal region:** The human Y chromosome is composed of two different parts: a pseudoautosomal region that is homologous to a region of the X chromosome and which is responsible for sex chromosome pairing and a Y-specific part that encodes the sex-determining gene and a few other genes. Genes within the pseudoautosomal region are not sex-linked.

Reciprocal translocation:* A segment of one chromosome is exchanged with a segment of another chromosome of a different homologous pair.

Robertsonian translocation:* The joining of two acrocentric chromosomes at the centromeres with loss of their short arms to form a single abnormal chromosome; acrocentric chromosomes are chromosome numbers 13, 14, 15, 21, and 22.

Situs inversus: A complete reversal of the positions of the thoracic and abdominal organs resulting in a mirror image of the normal positioning, which is known as situs solitus.

Somatic cells:** All the body cells except the reproductive (germ) cells.

SRY gene: Sex-determining region of the Y chromosome.

Teratogen: A substance or agent which disturbs normal development of the embryo or fetus.

Trans configuration:* Term which indicates that an individual who is heterozygous at two neighboring loci has one of the mutations on one of two homologous chromosomes and the other on the other homolog.

Triallelic inheritance: A phenotype which results from three mutations in genes at two different loci.

Trinucleotide repeat:* Sequences of three nucleotides repeated in tandem on the same chromosome a number of times. A normal, polymorphic variation in repeat number with no clinical significance commonly occurs between individuals; however, repeat numbers over a certain threshold can, in some cases, lead to adverse effects on the function of the gene, resulting in genetic disease.

Trisomy:* The presence of a single extra chromosome, yielding a total of three chromosomes of that particular type instead of a pair. Partial trisomy refers to the presence of an extra copy of a segment of a chromosome.

Trisomy rescue:* The phenomenon in which a fertilized ovum initially contains 47 chromosomes (i.e., is trisomic), but loses one of the trisomic chromosomes in the process of cell division such that the resulting daughter cells and their descendants contain 46 chromosomes, the normal number.

Tumor suppressor gene:** Genes in the body that can suppress or block the development of cancer.

Uniparental disomy (UPD):* The situation in which both members of a chromosome pair or segments of a chromosome pair are inherited from one parent and neither is inherited from the other parent. Uniparental disomy can result in an abnormal phenotype in some cases.

Uniparental heterodisomy: Uniparental disomy with both members of a homologous pair of chromosomes from the same parent; the two members are not identical but instead are the two homologs present in the parent.

Uniparental isodisomy: Uniparental disomy with two identical copies of the same chromosome; the two copies represent only one of the parent's homologous pair.

Variable expression:* Variation in clinical features (type and severity) of a genetic disorder between individuals with the same gene alteration, even within the same family.

Wild type:\# The form of an organism that occurs most frequently in nature.

X-chromosome inactivation:* The phenomenon by which one X chromosome in females (either maternally or paternally derived) is randomly inactivated in early embryonic cells, with fixed inactivation in all descendant cells.

Zygote: The resulting cell when two gametes unite.

Sources

*   *GeneTests: Medical Genetics Information Resource* (database online). Educational Materials: Glossary in GeneTests. Copyright, University of Washington, Seattle. 1993–2009. Available at http://www.genetests.org. Accessed September 2009.

**   *Unified Medical Language System* (NCI Thesaurus) at the National Library of Medicine. www.cancer.gov.

***   *Talking Glossary of Genetic Terms* from the National Human Genome Research Institute.

\#   Human Genome Project Information. U.S Department of Energy Office of Science, Office of Biological and Environmental Research, Human Genome Program. www.ornl.gov/hgmis.

Index

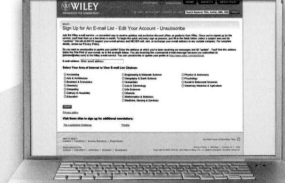
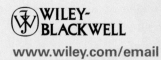